PAST
F

MCQs IN CARDIOLOGY AND RESPIRATORY MEDICINE

Edited by Richard L. Hawkins MBBS FRCS

Authors: Peter Wilmshurst MB ChB MRCP
St Thomas' Hospital, London.

John Moore-Gillon MA MD MRCP
The London Chest Hospital.

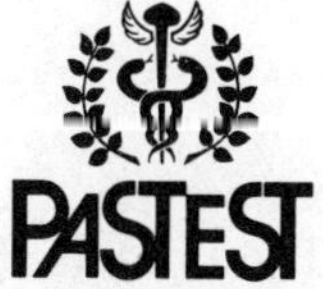

Rankin House, Parkgate Estate,
Knutsford, Cheshire. WA16 8DX

First printed 1987
Reprinted 1988
Reprinted 1989
Reprinted 1991
Reprinted 1993

A catalogue record for this book is available from the British Library.

ISBN: 0 906896 18 5

Text prepared by Turner Associates, Knutsford, Cheshire.
Phototypeset by Communitype, Leicester
Printed by Martins The Printers, Berwick on Tweed

CONTENTS

INTRODUCTION

With more than twelve years of experience in postgraduate medical education to draw on, PASTEST have commissioned a series of reasonably priced MCQ books under the editorial mantle of Dr Richard Hawkins.

There is no better way to revise for the MRCP Part I examination than by answering good quality MCQs. These books, however, provide an additional dimension. The MCQs have been deliberately broken down by specialty and a self-assessment chart provided for each so that doctors can identify their strengths and weaknesses and plan their revision accordingly.

A significant number of questions in the MRCP Part I examination are devoted to Cardiology. and Respiratory Medicine. This book provides 50 representative questions from each specialty, with each question accompanied by a clear and simple explanatory answer. A strong emphasis on physiology, basic sciences and pharmacology has been included since the modern examination places such importance on these aspects.

The membership examination at present consists of sixty questions, each with a stem and five related questions: a total of 300 possible correct responses. Each correct response is awarded +1, each incorrect one -1, with no marks being awarded if the question is answered 'Don't know'. As in all examinations proper technique can make the difference between a 'pass' and a 'bare fail'.

What, then, is the best approach? Firstly, the question stem must be read very carefully. Failure to notice a negative statement could result in a score of -5. In a 'close marked' examination this could quite easily be the difference between a pass and a fail. Secondly, the keywords used in MCQs should be identified; always/commonly/frequently/recognised/may/never, and so on. Each has a distinctly different meaning, thus: 'jaundice is a frequent complication of infectious mononucleosis' (false), whereas: 'jaundice may complicate infectious mononucleosis' (true). Beware of always and never.

Finally, answer those questions that you think you have a greater than 50% chance of getting correct. Thus, while leaving out questions in which you would be guessing (because in these you are likely to score 0 overall), do attempt those which you think you know something about; it is worth backing a hunch. Although your 'hit rate' will not be as high for these as for those questions for which you think you know the answer, overall you will score positively. Candidates do fail because they do not attempt enough questions, and it is worth remembering that even some of those answers that you are confident about may, in fact, be wrong.

Time for revision is often at a premium because preparation has to be done at the same time as a busy medical SHO job. A few general tips may be useful:

1. Do not read systematically through large medical textbooks, but rather base your revision around multiple choice questions. The self-assessment charts provided in this book may be helpful here. Direct further reading of standard texts to those areas in which you are scoring low marks, in other words use these MCQs to identify 'blind spots' in your knowledge.

2. Make cards for those questions which come up frequently (such as modes of inheritance) and learn these.

3. A good course is probably worth the investment and your employer may be able to assist with the funding for this, if one is not provided at your hospital.

4. Aim to start your revision in good time and be sure you have time to cover most topics.

Two cut-out self-assessment charts are included in this book so that you can record your answers to each MCQ as you work steadily through the questions. In order to give yourself a realistic time limit, do not spend more than 2 ½ minutes on any one question. Some people may prefer to indicate their answers directly on the question pages in the spaces provided and then to transfer these answers on to the self-assessment charts. You can then correct your own answers against the answers given in the book and can calculate your total score in each section. By indicating clearly each item that you answered incorrectly you can then read the explanation provided and refer to a standard text book for further revision on that topic.

Encyclopaedic specialist reference books are perhaps best avoided during preparation, only to be used for verification of detail. There is a plethora of books on clinical electrocardiography, both Shamroth's **An Introduction to Electrocardiography** (Blackwell, Oxford), and P. S. Burge's **ECGs for Examinations** (Lloyd Luke), being excellent. Lung function is well covered by both **Pulmonary Pathophysiology** by West (Williams and Wilkins, London) and **Lung Function for the Clinician** by Hughes and Empey (Academic Press, London).

CARDIOLOGY SELF-ASSESSMENT CHART

Please use 2B PENCIL only. Rub out all errors thoroughly.
Mark lozenges like ⬬ NOT like this ⊄ ⊄ ⊄

T ⬭ = TRUE F ⬭ = FALSE DK ⬭ = DON'T KNOW

	A	B	C	D	E
1	T ⬭ F ⬭ DK ⬭	T ⬭ F ⬭ DK ⬭	T ⬭ F ⬭ DK ⬭	T ⬭ F ⬭ DK ⬭	T ⬭ F ⬭ DK ⬭
2	T ⬭ F ⬭ DK ⬭	T ⬭ F ⬭ DK ⬭	T ⬭ F ⬭ DK ⬭	T ⬭ F ⬭ DK ⬭	T ⬭ F ⬭ DK ⬭
3	T ⬭ F ⬭ DK ⬭	T ⬭ F ⬭ DK ⬭	T ⬭ F ⬭ DK ⬭	T ⬭ F ⬭ DK ⬭	T ⬭ F ⬭ DK ⬭
4	T ⬭ F ⬭ DK ⬭	T ⬭ F ⬭ DK ⬭	T ⬭ F ⬭ DK ⬭	T ⬭ F ⬭ DK ⬭	T ⬭ F ⬭ DK ⬭
5	T ⬭ F ⬭ DK ⬭	T ⬭ F ⬭ DK ⬭	T ⬭ F ⬭ DK ⬭	T ⬭ F ⬭ DK ⬭	T ⬭ F ⬭ DK ⬭
6	T ⬭ F ⬭ DK ⬭	T ⬭ F ⬭ DK ⬭	T ⬭ F ⬭ DK ⬭	T ⬭ F ⬭ DK ⬭	T ⬭ F ⬭ DK ⬭
7	T ⬭ F ⬭ DK ⬭	T ⬭ F ⬭ DK ⬭	T ⬭ F ⬭ DK ⬭	T ⬭ F ⬭ DK ⬭	T ⬭ F ⬭ DK ⬭
8	T ⬭ F ⬭ DK ⬭	T ⬭ F ⬭ DK ⬭	T ⬭ F ⬭ DK ⬭	T ⬭ F ⬭ DK ⬭	T ⬭ F ⬭ DK ⬭
9	T ⬭ F ⬭ DK ⬭	T ⬭ F ⬭ DK ⬭	T ⬭ F ⬭ DK ⬭	T ⬭ F ⬭ DK ⬭	T ⬭ F ⬭ DK ⬭
10	T ⬭ F ⬭ DK ⬭	T ⬭ F ⬭ DK ⬭	T ⬭ F ⬭ DK ⬭	T ⬭ F ⬭ DK ⬭	T ⬭ F ⬭ DK ⬭
11	T ⬭ F ⬭ DK ⬭	T ⬭ F ⬭ DK ⬭	T ⬭ F ⬭ DK ⬭	T ⬭ F ⬭ DK ⬭	T ⬭ F ⬭ DK ⬭
12	T ⬭ F ⬭ DK ⬭	T ⬭ F ⬭ DK ⬭	T ⬭ F ⬭ DK ⬭	T ⬭ F ⬭ DK ⬭	T ⬭ F ⬭ DK ⬭
13	T ⬭ F ⬭ DK ⬭	T ⬭ F ⬭ DK ⬭	T ⬭ F ⬭ DK ⬭	T ⬭ F ⬭ DK ⬭	T ⬭ F ⬭ DK ⬭
14	T ⬭ F ⬭ DK ⬭	T ⬭ F ⬭ DK ⬭	T ⬭ F ⬭ DK ⬭	T ⬭ F ⬭ DK ⬭	T ⬭ F ⬭ DK ⬭
15	T ⬭ F ⬭ DK ⬭	T ⬭ F ⬭ DK ⬭	T ⬭ F ⬭ DK ⬭	T ⬭ F ⬭ DK ⬭	T ⬭ F ⬭ DK ⬭

	A	B	C	D	E
16	T ⬭ F ⬭ DK ⬭	T ⬭ F ⬭ DK ⬭	T ⬭ F ⬭ DK ⬭	T ⬭ F ⬭ DK ⬭	T ⬭ F ⬭ DK ⬭
17	T ⬭ F ⬭ DK ⬭	T ⬭ F ⬭ DK ⬭	T ⬭ F ⬭ DK ⬭	T ⬭ F ⬭ DK ⬭	T ⬭ F ⬭ DK ⬭
18	T ⬭ F ⬭ DK ⬭	T ⬭ F ⬭ DK ⬭	T ⬭ F ⬭ DK ⬭	T ⬭ F ⬭ DK ⬭	T ⬭ F ⬭ DK ⬭
19	T ⬭ F ⬭ DK ⬭	T ⬭ F ⬭ DK ⬭	T ⬭ F ⬭ DK ⬭	T ⬭ F ⬭ DK ⬭	T ⬭ F ⬭ DK ⬭
20	T ⬭ F ⬭ DK ⬭	T ⬭ F ⬭ DK ⬭	T ⬭ F ⬭ DK ⬭	T ⬭ F ⬭ DK ⬭	T ⬭ F ⬭ DK ⬭
21	T ⬭ F ⬭ DK ⬭	T ⬭ F ⬭ DK ⬭	T ⬭ F ⬭ DK ⬭	T ⬭ F ⬭ DK ⬭	T ⬭ F ⬭ DK ⬭
22	T ⬭ F ⬭ DK ⬭	T ⬭ F ⬭ DK ⬭	T ⬭ F ⬭ DK ⬭	T ⬭ F ⬭ DK ⬭	T ⬭ F ⬭ DK ⬭
23	T ⬭ F ⬭ DK ⬭	T ⬭ F ⬭ DK ⬭	T ⬭ F ⬭ DK ⬭	T ⬭ F ⬭ DK ⬭	T ⬭ F ⬭ DK ⬭
24	T ⬭ F ⬭ DK ⬭	T ⬭ F ⬭ DK ⬭	T ⬭ F ⬭ DK ⬭	T ⬭ F ⬭ DK ⬭	T ⬭ F ⬭ DK ⬭
25	T ⬭ F ⬭ DK ⬭	T ⬭ F ⬭ DK ⬭	T ⬭ F ⬭ DK ⬭	T ⬭ F ⬭ DK ⬭	T ⬭ F ⬭ DK ⬭
26	T ⬭ F ⬭ DK ⬭	T ⬭ F ⬭ DK ⬭	T ⬭ F ⬭ DK ⬭	T ⬭ F ⬭ DK ⬭	T ⬭ F ⬭ DK ⬭
27	T ⬭ F ⬭ DK ⬭	T ⬭ F ⬭ DK ⬭	T ⬭ F ⬭ DK ⬭	T ⬭ F ⬭ DK ⬭	T ⬭ F ⬭ DK ⬭
28	T ⬭ F ⬭ DK ⬭	T ⬭ F ⬭ DK ⬭	T ⬭ F ⬭ DK ⬭	T ⬭ F ⬭ DK ⬭	T ⬭ F ⬭ DK ⬭
29	T ⬭ F ⬭ DK ⬭	T ⬭ F ⬭ DK ⬭	T ⬭ F ⬭ DK ⬭	T ⬭ F ⬭ DK ⬭	T ⬭ F ⬭ DK ⬭
30	T ⬭ F ⬭ DK ⬭	T ⬭ F ⬭ DK ⬭	T ⬭ F ⬭ DK ⬭	T ⬭ F ⬭ DK ⬭	T ⬭ F ⬭ DK ⬭

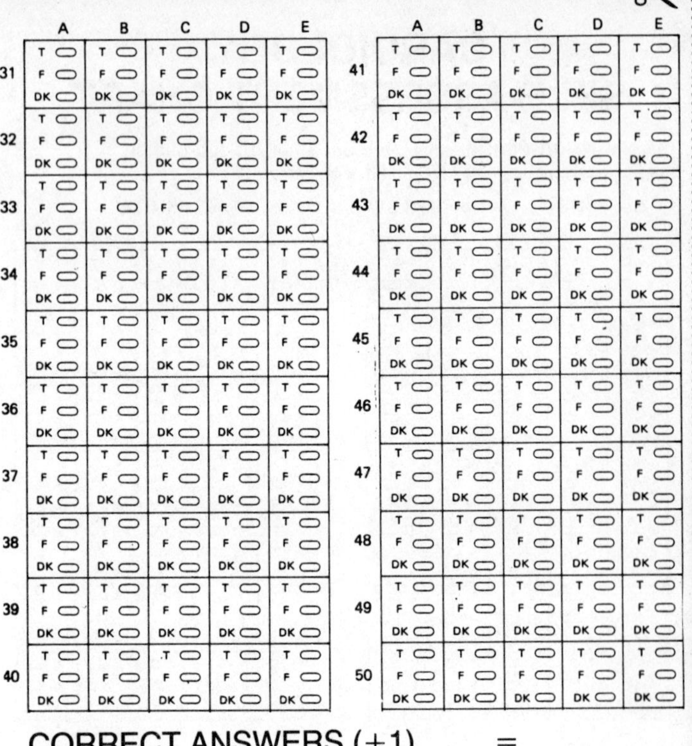

	A	B	C	D	E
31	T F DK	T F DK	T F DK	T F DK	T F DK
32	T F DK	T F DK	T F DK	T F DK	T F DK
33	T F DK	T F DK	T F DK	T F DK	T F DK
34	T F DK	T F DK	T F DK	T F DK	T F DK
35	T F DK	T F DK	T F DK	T F DK	T F DK
36	T F DK	T F DK	T F DK	T F DK	T F DK
37	T F DK	T F DK	T F DK	T F DK	T F DK
38	T F DK	T F DK	T F DK	T F DK	T F DK
39	T F DK	T F DK	T F DK	T F DK	T F DK
40	T F DK	T F DK	T F DK	T F DK	T F DK

	A	B	C	D	E
41	T F DK	T F DK	T F DK	T F DK	T F DK
42	T F DK	T F DK	T F DK	T F DK	T F DK
43	T F DK	T F DK	T F DK	T F DK	T F DK
44	T F DK	T F DK	T F DK	T F DK	T F DK
45	T F DK	T F DK	T F DK	T F DK	T F DK
46	T F DK	T F DK	T F DK	T F DK	T F DK
47	T F DK	T F DK	T F DK	T F DK	T F DK
48	T F DK	T F DK	T F DK	T F DK	T F DK
49	T F DK	T F DK	T F DK	T F DK	T F DK
50	T F DK	T F DK	T F DK	T F DK	T F DK

CORRECT ANSWERS (+1) =

INCORRECT ANSWERS (−1) =

DON'T KNOW (0) ______

TOTAL SCORE: ______

RESPIRATORY MEDICINE SELF-ASSESSMENT CHART

Please use 2B PENCIL only. Rub out all errors thoroughly.
Mark lozenges like ⬬ NOT like this ⊄ ⊄ ⊄

T ⬭ = TRUE F ⬭ = FALSE DK ⬭ = DON'T KNOW

	A	B	C	D	E
51	T ⬭ F ⬭ DK ⬭	T ⬭ F ⬭ DK ⬭	T ⬭ F ⬭ DK ⬭	T ⬭ F ⬭ DK ⬭	T ⬭ F ⬭ DK ⬭
52	T ⬭ F ⬭ DK ⬭	T ⬭ F ⬭ DK ⬭	T ⬭ F ⬭ DK ⬭	T ⬭ F ⬭ DK ⬭	T ⬭ F ⬭ DK ⬭
53	T ⬭ F ⬭ DK ⬭	T ⬭ F ⬭ DK ⬭	T ⬭ F ⬭ DK ⬭	T ⬭ F ⬭ DK ⬭	T ⬭ F ⬭ DK ⬭
54	T ⬭ F ⬭ DK ⬭	T ⬭ F ⬭ DK ⬭	T ⬭ F ⬭ DK ⬭	T ⬭ F ⬭ DK ⬭	T ⬭ F ⬭ DK ⬭
55	T ⬭ F ⬭ DK ⬭	T ⬭ F ⬭ DK ⬭	T ⬭ F ⬭ DK ⬭	T ⬭ F ⬭ DK ⬭	T ⬭ F ⬭ DK ⬭
56	T ⬭ F ⬭ DK ⬭	T ⬭ F ⬭ DK ⬭	T ⬭ F ⬭ DK ⬭	T ⬭ F ⬭ DK ⬭	T ⬭ F ⬭ DK ⬭
57	T ⬭ F ⬭ DK ⬭	T ⬭ F ⬭ DK ⬭	T ⬭ F ⬭ DK ⬭	T ⬭ F ⬭ DK ⬭	T ⬭ F ⬭ DK ⬭
58	T ⬭ F ⬭ DK ⬭	T ⬭ F ⬭ DK ⬭	T ⬭ F ⬭ DK ⬭	T ⬭ F ⬭ DK ⬭	T ⬭ F ⬭ DK ⬭
59	T ⬭ F ⬭ DK ⬭	T ⬭ F ⬭ DK ⬭	T ⬭ F ⬭ DK ⬭	T ⬭ F ⬭ DK ⬭	T ⬭ F ⬭ DK ⬭
60	T ⬭ F ⬭ DK ⬭	T ⬭ F ⬭ DK ⬭	T ⬭ F ⬭ DK ⬭	T ⬭ F ⬭ DK ⬭	T ⬭ F ⬭ DK ⬭
61	T ⬭ F ⬭ DK ⬭	T ⬭ F ⬭ DK ⬭	T ⬭ F ⬭ DK ⬭	T ⬭ F ⬭ DK ⬭	T ⬭ F ⬭ DK ⬭
62	T ⬭ F ⬭ DK ⬭	T ⬭ F ⬭ DK ⬭	T ⬭ F ⬭ DK ⬭	T ⬭ F ⬭ DK ⬭	T ⬭ F ⬭ DK ⬭
63	T ⬭ F ⬭ DK ⬭	T ⬭ F ⬭ DK ⬭	T ⬭ F ⬭ DK ⬭	T ⬭ F ⬭ DK ⬭	T ⬭ F ⬭ DK ⬭
64	T ⬭ F ⬭ DK ⬭	T ⬭ F ⬭ DK ⬭	T ⬭ F ⬭ DK ⬭	T ⬭ F ⬭ DK ⬭	T ⬭ F ⬭ DK ⬭
65	T ⬭ F ⬭ DK ⬭	T ⬭ F ⬭ DK ⬭	T ⬭ F ⬭ DK ⬭	T ⬭ F ⬭ DK ⬭	T ⬭ F ⬭ DK ⬭
66	T ⬭ F ⬭ DK ⬭	T ⬭ F ⬭ DK ⬭	T ⬭ F ⬭ DK ⬭	T ⬭ F ⬭ DK ⬭	T ⬭ F ⬭ DK ⬭
67	T ⬭ F ⬭ DK ⬭	T ⬭ F ⬭ DK ⬭	T ⬭ F ⬭ DK ⬭	T ⬭ F ⬭ DK ⬭	T ⬭ F ⬭ DK ⬭
68	T ⬭ F ⬭ DK ⬭	T ⬭ F ⬭ DK ⬭	T ⬭ F ⬭ DK ⬭	T ⬭ F ⬭ DK ⬭	T ⬭ F ⬭ DK ⬭
69	T ⬭ F ⬭ DK ⬭	T ⬭ F ⬭ DK ⬭	T ⬭ F ⬭ DK ⬭	T ⬭ F ⬭ DK ⬭	T ⬭ F ⬭ DK ⬭
70	T ⬭ F ⬭ DK ⬭	T ⬭ F ⬭ DK ⬭	T ⬭ F ⬭ DK ⬭	T ⬭ F ⬭ DK ⬭	T ⬭ F ⬭ DK ⬭
71	T ⬭ F ⬭ DK ⬭	T ⬭ F ⬭ DK ⬭	T ⬭ F ⬭ DK ⬭	T ⬭ F ⬭ DK ⬭	T ⬭ F ⬭ DK ⬭
72	T ⬭ F ⬭ DK ⬭	T ⬭ F ⬭ DK ⬭	T ⬭ F ⬭ DK ⬭	T ⬭ F ⬭ DK ⬭	T ⬭ F ⬭ DK ⬭
73	T ⬭ F ⬭ DK ⬭	T ⬭ F ⬭ DK ⬭	T ⬭ F ⬭ DK ⬭	T ⬭ F ⬭ DK ⬭	T ⬭ F ⬭ DK ⬭
74	T ⬭ F ⬭ DK ⬭	T ⬭ F ⬭ DK ⬭	T ⬭ F ⬭ DK ⬭	T ⬭ F ⬭ DK ⬭	T ⬭ F ⬭ DK ⬭
75	T ⬭ F ⬭ DK ⬭	T ⬭ F ⬭ DK ⬭	T ⬭ F ⬭ DK ⬭	T ⬭ F ⬭ DK ⬭	T ⬭ F ⬭ DK ⬭
76	T ⬭ F ⬭ DK ⬭	T ⬭ F ⬭ DK ⬭	T ⬭ F ⬭ DK ⬭	T ⬭ F ⬭ DK ⬭	T ⬭ F ⬭ DK ⬭
77	T ⬭ F ⬭ DK ⬭	T ⬭ F ⬭ DK ⬭	T ⬭ F ⬭ DK ⬭	T ⬭ F ⬭ DK ⬭	T ⬭ F ⬭ DK ⬭
78	T ⬭ F ⬭ DK ⬭	T ⬭ F ⬭ DK ⬭	T ⬭ F ⬭ DK ⬭	T ⬭ F ⬭ DK ⬭	T ⬭ F ⬭ DK ⬭
79	T ⬭ F ⬭ DK ⬭	T ⬭ F ⬭ DK ⬭	T ⬭ F ⬭ DK ⬭	T ⬭ F ⬭ DK ⬭	T ⬭ F ⬭ DK ⬭
80	T ⬭ F ⬭ DK ⬭	T ⬭ F ⬭ DK ⬭	T ⬭ F ⬭ DK ⬭	T ⬭ F ⬭ DK ⬭	T ⬭ F ⬭ DK ⬭

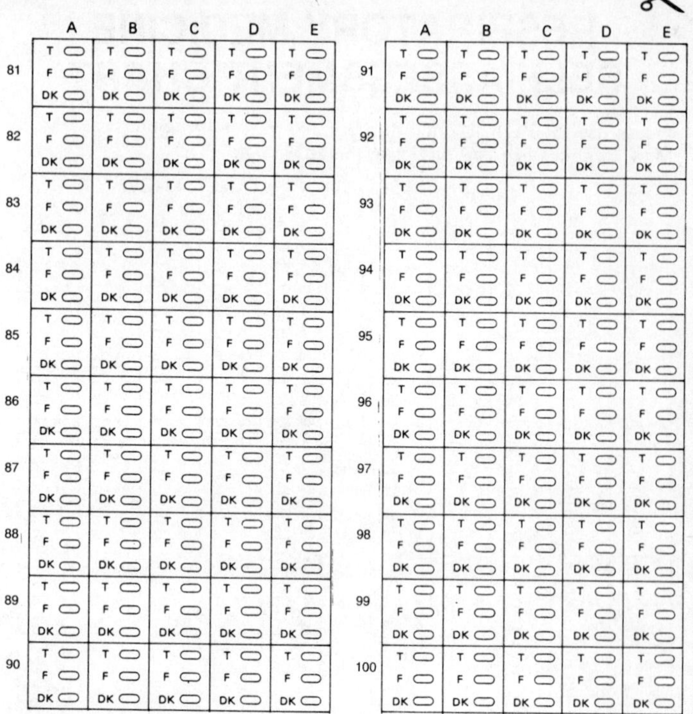

	A	B	C	D	E
81	T ⬭ F ⬭ DK ⬭	T ⬭ F ⬭ DK ⬭	T ⬭ F ⬭ DK ⬭	T ⬭ F ⬭ DK ⬭	T ⬭ F ⬭ DK ⬭
82	T ⬭ F ⬭ DK ⬭	T ⬭ F ⬭ DK ⬭	T ⬭ F ⬭ DK ⬭	T ⬭ F ⬭ DK ⬭	T ⬭ F ⬭ DK ⬭
83	T ⬭ F ⬭ DK ⬭	T ⬭ F ⬭ DK ⬭	T ⬭ F ⬭ DK ⬭	T ⬭ F ⬭ DK ⬭	T ⬭ F ⬭ DK ⬭
84	T ⬭ F ⬭ DK ⬭	T ⬭ F ⬭ DK ⬭	T ⬭ F ⬭ DK ⬭	T ⬭ F ⬭ DK ⬭	T ⬭ F ⬭ DK ⬭
85	T ⬭ F ⬭ DK ⬭	T ⬭ F ⬭ DK ⬭	T ⬭ F ⬭ DK ⬭	T ⬭ F ⬭ DK ⬭	T ⬭ F ⬭ DK ⬭
86	T ⬭ F ⬭ DK ⬭	T ⬭ F ⬭ DK ⬭	T ⬭ F ⬭ DK ⬭	T ⬭ F ⬭ DK ⬭	T ⬭ F ⬭ DK ⬭
87	T ⬭ F ⬭ DK ⬭	T ⬭ F ⬭ DK ⬭	T ⬭ F ⬭ DK ⬭	T ⬭ F ⬭ DK ⬭	T ⬭ F ⬭ DK ⬭
88	T ⬭ F ⬭ DK ⬭	T ⬭ F ⬭ DK ⬭	T ⬭ F ⬭ DK ⬭	T ⬭ F ⬭ DK ⬭	T ⬭ F ⬭ DK ⬭
89	T ⬭ F ⬭ DK ⬭	T ⬭ F ⬭ DK ⬭	T ⬭ F ⬭ DK ⬭	T ⬭ F ⬭ DK ⬭	T ⬭ F ⬭ DK ⬭
90	T ⬭ F ⬭ DK ⬭	T ⬭ F ⬭ DK ⬭	T ⬭ F ⬭ DK ⬭	T ⬭ F ⬭ DK ⬭	T ⬭ F ⬭ DK ⬭

	A	B	C	D	E
91	T ⬭ F ⬭ DK ⬭	T ⬭ F ⬭ DK ⬭	T ⬭ F ⬭ DK ⬭	T ⬭ F ⬭ DK ⬭	T ⬭ F ⬭ DK ⬭
92	T ⬭ F ⬭ DK ⬭	T ⬭ F ⬭ DK ⬭	T ⬭ F ⬭ DK ⬭	T ⬭ F ⬭ DK ⬭	T ⬭ F ⬭ DK ⬭
93	T ⬭ F ⬭ DK ⬭	T ⬭ F ⬭ DK ⬭	T ⬭ F ⬭ DK ⬭	T ⬭ F ⬭ DK ⬭	T ⬭ F ⬭ DK ⬭
94	T ⬭ F ⬭ DK ⬭	T ⬭ F ⬭ DK ⬭	T ⬭ F ⬭ DK ⬭	T ⬭ F ⬭ DK ⬭	T ⬭ F ⬭ DK ⬭
95	T ⬭ F ⬭ DK ⬭	T ⬭ F ⬭ DK ⬭	T ⬭ F ⬭ DK ⬭	T ⬭ F ⬭ DK ⬭	T ⬭ F ⬭ DK ⬭
96	T ⬭ F ⬭ DK ⬭	T ⬭ F ⬭ DK ⬭	T ⬭ F ⬭ DK ⬭	T ⬭ F ⬭ DK ⬭	T ⬭ F ⬭ DK ⬭
97	T ⬭ F ⬭ DK ⬭	T ⬭ F ⬭ DK ⬭	T ⬭ F ⬭ DK ⬭	T ⬭ F ⬭ DK ⬭	T ⬭ F ⬭ DK ⬭
98	T ⬭ F ⬭ DK ⬭	T ⬭ F ⬭ DK ⬭	T ⬭ F ⬭ DK ⬭	T ⬭ F ⬭ DK ⬭	T ⬭ F ⬭ DK ⬭
99	T ⬭ F ⬭ DK ⬭	T ⬭ F ⬭ DK ⬭	T ⬭ F ⬭ DK ⬭	T ⬭ F ⬭ DK ⬭	T ⬭ F ⬭ DK ⬭
100	T ⬭ F ⬭ DK ⬭	T ⬭ F ⬭ DK ⬭	T ⬭ F ⬭ DK ⬭	T ⬭ F ⬭ DK ⬭	T ⬭ F ⬭ DK ⬭

CORRECT ANSWERS (+1) =

INCORRECT ANSWERS (−1) =

DON'T KNOW (0) __________

TOTAL SCORE: __________

CARDIOLOGY

Indicate your answers by putting T (True), F (False) or D (Don't know) in the spaces provided.

1. Ventricular septal defects

A do not produce right atrial volume overload unless a Gerbode defect is present
B may be complicated by infective endocarditis no matter how small the defect
C do not produce the Eisenmenger syndrome until adult life
D usually affect the muscular part of the septum
E are characterised by a systolic murmur at the sternal edge and right bundle branch block on the electrocardiogram

Your answers: A.........B.........C.........D.........E.........

2. In Fallot's tetralogy

A cyanosis is characteristically present, but may not be detected at birth
B the second heart sound is widely split
C the chest X-ray shows plethoric lung fields
D cerebral abscesses occur because of right to left shunting of blood in the heart
E pulmonary hypertension develops in early life

Your answers: A.........B.........C.........D.........E.........

3. Coarctation of the aorta is

A usually congenital but may be acquired
B recognised by absent or delayed femoral artery pulses
C a common cause of heart failure in infancy but an uncommon cause of hypertension in adults
D associated with an increased incidence of bicuspid aortic valve
E a cause of left to right shunting of blood

Your answers: A.........B.........C.........D.........E.........

Answers overleaf

ANSWERS AND EXPLANATIONS

1. A B

Ventricular septal defects usually involve the membranous septum. A Gerbode defect occurs when the defect passes between the left ventricle and the right atrium and it occurs because the mitral valve is normally attached to the interventricular septum higher than the tricuspid valve. Pulmonary hypertension and the Eisenmenger syndrome can occur at an early age if the defect is large. Right bundle branch block is more characteristic of atrial septal defects and the electrocardiogram seen in patients with ventricular septal defects may vary from normal to gross ventricular hypertrophy.

2. A D

The features of Fallot's tetralogy are due to a combination of a ventricular septal defect and pulmonary stenosis. This causes shunting of blood from the right to left ventricles, which results in cyanosis. However, in mild cases, cyanosis does not develop until a day or two after birth, when the ductus arteriosus closes. The presence of the right to left shunt also causes diversion of blood away from the lungs, which appear oligaemic on chest X-ray and can result in cerebral abscesses. The presence of pulmonary stenosis protects against development of pulmonary hypertension. The second heart sound is single.

3. A B C D

A coarctation is narrowing or obliteration of the aortic lumen. It may be acquired but is usually congenital, when it is most commonly situated just distal to the origin of the left subclavian artery. Coarctation of the aorta is the commonest cause of heart failure in babies who are not cyanosed and is an uncommon cause of hypertension in adult life. Coarctation is associated with other cardiac abnormalities, particularly bicuspid aortic valve, but does not itself cause cardiac shunting. Coarctation is recognised by absent or delayed pulses in the legs compared with those in the arms.

4. In a patient with an atrial septal defect

A left axis deviation on the electrocardiogram suggests a secundum defect

B the presence of anomalous right pulmonary venous drainage into the right atrium suggests a sinus venosus defect

C a tricuspid diastolic murmur suggests a large left to right shunt

D sinus arrhythmia is present if the shunt is large

E symptoms may only develop in middle age

Your answers: A.........B.........C.........D.........E.........

5. Transposition of the great arteries

A is not compatible with survival unless a septal defect, persistent ductus arteriosus or atrioventricular discordance is also present

B typically does not produce cyanosis in infancy

C typically does not produce heart failure in infancy

D occurs when the aorta develops posteriorly to the pulmonary trunk

E characteristically is complicated by tricuspid valve regurgitation

Your answers: A........B.........C........D.........E.........

6. In the newborn infant the following circulatory changes occur:

A peripheral vascular resistance rises

B pulmonary vascular resistance rises

C blood flow across the foramen ovale reverses

D blood flow across the ductus arteriosus is initially reduced and reversed immediately after birth before ceasing entirely in a further day or two

E superior vena caval blood flow exceeds inferior vena caval blood flow for the first time

Your answers: A........B........C........D........E........

Answers overleaf

4. B C E

In a patient with an atrial septal defect, right axis deviation suggests a secundum defect (most common type) and left axis deviation suggests a primum defect (less common). Sinus venosus defects are the least common type of defect and are frequently associated with anomalous right pulmonary venous drainage. Sinus arrhythmia is only present in patients with small defects and a tricuspid flow murmur suggests a large shunt. Pulmonary hypertension is a late feature of atrial septal defects and symptoms may only develop in middle age.

5. A E

In transposition of the great arteries the aorta arises from the right ventricle and hence anteriorly to the pulmonary artery which arises from the left ventricle. The condition is incompatible with extrauterine survival, unless a shunt is present or atrioventricular discordance results in 'corrected transposition'. Typically death in infancy due to heart failure and cyanosis occurs. If longer term survival occurs, a significant complication is tricuspid regurgitation due to the abnormally high (systemic) pressures generated by the right ventricle.

6. A D E

After birth, the lungs inflate which causes pulmonary vascular resistance to fall. In utero, the placental vessels cause the systemic vascular resistance to be low and inferior vena caval flow to be high. When placental blood flow ceases, the systemic vascular resistance rises and for the first time superior vena caval flow exceeds inferior vena caval flow. Also at birth the foramen ovale closes (rather like a flap) as left atrial pressure and lung blood flow increase. The ductus arteriosus narrows at birth but does not close for a day or two. During those initial days, the direction of flow across the ductus arteriosus is reversed since the high pulmonary vascular resistance and low systemic vascular resistance present in utero are reversed.

7. During the normal cardiac cycle

A initial myocardial depolarisation occurs at a site near to the junction of the right atrium and inferior vena cava

B there is no time when all cardiac chambers are simultaneously in diastole

C the dicrotic notch of the aortic pressure trace coincides with the second heart sound

D a third heart sound is never heard

E the majority of coronary artery flow occurs during ventricular diastole

Your answers: A.........B.........C.........D.........E.........

8. During the normal cardiac cycle

A the aortic and pulmonary valves close synchronously

B the period of left ventricular isovolumic contraction occurs between the first heart sound and the onset of the carotid upstroke

C the v wave of the jugular venous pulse coincides with the carotid pulse

D the interventricular septum depolarises from right to left

E right ventricular systole is prolonged during expiration

Your answers: A.........B.........C.........D.........E.........

9. The following statements are correct:

A stimulation of the right vagus nerve slows the rate of sinus node depolarisation whilst stimulation of the left vagus nerve delays atrioventricular conduction

B stimulation of either phrenic nerve produces a sinus tachycardia

C blood in the coronary sinus has a very low oxygen content at all times, irrespective of the level of activity of the individual

D the heart responds to increased myocardial oxygen requirements by coronary dilatation

E hyperbaric oxygen increases coronary vascular resistance

Your answers: A.........B.........C.........D.........E.........

Answers overleaf

7. C E

The cardiac cycle is initiated by depolarisation of the sinus node which is situated in the right atrium near the superior vena cava. Immediately prior to sinus node depolarisation all cardiac chambers are in diastole. It is during ventricular diastole that coronary flow occurs since this is the only time when aortic pressure exceeds left ventricular wall tension. Ventricular diastole extends from the closure of the aortic valve and hence the second heart sound and the aortic dicrotic notch to the subsequent ventricular depolarisation. During diastole, a third sound may be heard when ventricular filling is rapid. Generally a third heart sound is pathological, but may be also heard in young, fit individuals.

8. B

Depolarisation and contraction of the left and right ventricles are not precisely simultaneous. The initial ventricular depolarisation occurs in the septum and spreads from left to right. The aortic valve closes before the pulmonary valve, and the splitting of the second heart sound which results is accentuated during inspiration when right ventricular filling is increased and contraction is prolonged. Left ventricular isovolumic contraction occurs between closure of the mitral valve (first heart sound) and opening of aortic valve (carotid upstroke). The carotid pulse precedes the v wave of the jugular venous pulse.

9. A C D E

The vagus nerves supply parasympathetic innervation to the heart. The right vagus innervates the sinus node and the left innervates the atrioventricular node. The phrenic nerves lie either side of the heart and may be damaged during cardiac surgery, but innervate the diaphragms not the heart. The coronary vessels dilate when myocardial oxygen requirements increase and constrict if the oxygen content of blood is increased. The myocardial venous blood, which drains largely into the coronary sinus, always has a very low oxygen content because of high myocardial oxygen extraction.

10. The following statements are correct for cardiac muscle:

A cardiac muscle differs from smooth and striated muscle because of its inherent rhythmicity
B depolarisation of cardiac muscle is the result of an initial calcium influx
C repolarisation of cardiac muscle is the result of potassium efflux
D calcium ions are required for electromechanical coupling of the cardiac myosite
E the energy for contraction of the cardiac myosite is provided as adenosine diphosphate

Your answers: A.........B.........C.........D.........E.........

11. The following metabolic and neurohumoral effects are observed in patients with congestive cardiac failure:

A compensatory reduction in basal metabolic rate
B inhibition of aldosterone secretion because of sodium retention
C polycythaemia
D increased circulating renin concentrations
E increased responsiveness of the heart to circulating catecholamines

Your answers: A.........B.........C.........D.........E.........

12. During strenuous exercise in normal subjects

A the increase in cardiac output is mainly the result of increased stroke volume
B systolic and diastolic arterial pressures rise comparably
C skeletal muscle blood flow does not increase until the pH of muscle capillary blood starts to fall
D the vasodilatation of muscle blood vessels is counteracted by splanchnic vasoconstriction so that total peripheral vascular resistance is unaltered
E the arteriovenous oxygen difference falls

Your answers: A.........B.........C.........D.........E.........

Answers overleaf

10. A C D

Cardiac muscle contracts rhythmically, unlike other forms of muscle. However, like other types of muscle the myosites depolarise as a result of sodium influx and repolarise because of potassium efflux. Electromechanical coupling is dependent on calcium ions and adenosine triphosphate.

11. D

Neither the basal metabolic rate nor the oxygen carrying capacity of the blood is altered in congestive heart failure. Instead the body responds to reductions in blood pressure and cardiac output as if these were due to hypovolaemia. The resulting homoeostatic mechanisms are designed to increase circulating volume by retaining salt and water as well as raise blood pressure by vasoconstriction and inotropic stimulation of the heart. Changes include increased renin secretion and inappropriate aldosterone secretion (i.e. normal or raised aldosterone despite sodium retention). Circulating catecholamines are raised but cardiac responsiveness is decreased possibly due to receptor down regulation.

12. None of the answers is correct

During strenuous exercise the metabolic rate increases considerably. The increased tissue oxygen requirements are met by increased tissue oxygen extraction, which increases the arteriovenous oxygen difference, and an increase in cardiac output, which is mainly the result of an increase in heart rate and only a small increase in stroke volume. Systolic arterial pressure rises more than diastolic pressure. Muscle blood flow increases very considerably and although blood flow to inessential organs (e.g. splanchnic vessels) is reduced a little, the increased muscle blood flow causes peripheral vascular resistance to fall. The increase in muscle blood flow, like the increase in heart rate, occurs at the start of exercise before any measurable metabolic change can be detected.

13. On standing from the supine position

A compensatory changes in the circulation are the result of stimulation of carotid sinus and aortic baroreceptors by a reduced blood pressure

B reduced cerebral blood flow causes an increase in cerebral PCO_2 and a decrease in cerebral PO_2

C total peripheral vascular resistance decreases

D cardiac output increases

E circulating angiotensin II decreases

Your answers: A.........B.........C.........D.........E.........

14. The following statements about the Valsalva manoeuvre are correct:

A the manoeuvre is performed by straining to inhale against a closed glottis

B initially blood pressure increases transiently, then falls because venous return is impaired

C a tachycardia is present whilst straining but a bradycardia occurs after release of the manoeuvre

D the heart rate and blood pressure responses are abolished by sympathectomy

E the cardiovascular responses to the manoeuvre may be impaired in diabetes

Your answers: A.........B.........C.........D.........E.........

15. The physiological responses to haemorrhage include

A reduced discharge of afferent nerve fibres from the carotid sinus and aortic baroreceptors

B increased sympathetic activity because of activation of the vasomotor centre

C increased release of circulating atrial natriuretic peptide

D increased release of antidiuretic hormone

E increased glucocorticoid secretion

Your answers: A.........B.........C.........D.........E.........

Answers overleaf

13. A B

On standing from the supine position blood pools in the venous capacitance vessels of the legs. Cardiac output falls and total peripheral resistance increases. The arterial pressure at the level of the arterial baroreceptors is reduced and this stimulates compensatory changes. Homoeostatic mechanisms include increased angiotensin II secretion and sympathetic stimulation. On standing the arterial pressure in the cerebral vessels is reduced because these are now the highest part of the body. Cerebral blood flow is reduced and as a result the PCO_2 in brain tissue increases and the PO_2 decreases. These changes stimulate autoregulation of cerebral blood flow.

14. B C E

The Valsalva manoeuvre is performed by forced expiration against a closed glottis. The initial increase in intrathoracic pressure causes blood pressure to increase, but this soon falls because venous return is impaired. The fall in blood pressure is accompanied by a tachycardia and a rise in peripheral vascular resistance which are mediated through the baroreceptors. On release of the manoeuvre, venous return increases and hence blood pressure increases and in fact overshoots normal. This hypertension is accompanied by bradycardia. These cardiovascular effects persist after sympathectomy because the baroreceptors and vagi are intact. The responses can be impaired when autonomic neuropathy is present (e.g. in some diabetics).

15. A B D E

After haemorrhage and other hypovolaemic stresses, the arterial baroreceptors are stimulated. These have a tonic inhibitory effect on the vasomotor centre. As blood pressure falls the baroreceptors discharge less frequently and consequently the sympathetic efferents cause vasoconstriction and tachycardia. Baroreceptor stimulation also stimulates vasopressin (antidiuretic hormone) and ACTH release. Glucocorticoid concentrations in the blood are increased. Atrial natriuretic peptide secretion is reduced because blood volume is reduced and atrial stretch receptors are not activated.

16. The following statements are correct for Starling's law:

A the force of contraction is inversely proportional to the initial length of the cardiac muscle fibre
B the law is only true for isolated heart preparations
C the law means that stroke volume is proportional to left ventricular end diastolic volume unless the inotropic state of the myocardium or vascular resistance change
D as a consequence of the law, factors which reduce cardiac filling will increase contractility
E the law is dependent on the integrity of the cardiac stretch receptors

Your answers: A.........B.........C.........D.........E.........

17. The following factors cause arteriolar vasodilatation:

A raised PO_2
B raised PCO_2
C histamine
D serotonin
E raised local temperature

Your answers: A.........B.........C.........D.........E.........

18. A significant reduction in systemic arterial pressure is characteristically observed during inspiration in the following conditions:

A severe asthma attack
B positive pressure ventilation
C aortic dissection causing aortic regurgitation and cardiac tamponade
D massive pulmonary embolism
E massive haemorrhage

Your answers: A.........B.........C.........D.........E.........

Answers overleaf

16. B C

Starling's law states that in the isolated heart the force of contraction is directly proportional to the initial length of the cardiac fibre. When extrapolated to the whole animal, contractility and output impedance are also important determinants of stroke volume. However, generally factors which reduce cardiac filling also reduce stroke volume, but do not necessarily alter contractility. The law is dependent on the properties of myosites and the actin-myosin interaction. The cardiac stretch receptors do not play any part in Starling's law.

17. B C E

Arterioles dilate in response to increased local requirements which are manifest by metabolic changes such as decreased PO_2, increased PCO_2, reduced pH and increased local temperatures. A raised PO_2 is a vasoconstrictor stimulus. The highest concentrations of serotonin are present in platelets. Serotonin is released at the site of clot formation and causes vasoconstriction which has the effect of further reducing blood loss. Histamine is present in mast cells and released when trauma and allergic reactions occur. Histamine dilates arterioles but constricts veins.

18. A D E

Pulsus paradoxus is exaggeration of the normal slight fall in arterial pressure that occurs during inspiration and rise during expiration. Pulsus paradoxus occurs when greater than normal negative intra-thoracic pressures are generated during inspiration (e.g. asthma). When positive pressure ventilation is used, intrathoracic pressure is raised during inspiration so that blood pressure rises. Left ventricular underfilling is an important requirement for pulsus paradoxus and occurs in hypovolaemia and massive pulmonary embolism. Pulsus paradoxus also occurs in patients with cardiac tamponade, but when valvular lesions (e.g. aortic regurgitation) which prevent left ventricular underfilling are also present, pulsus paradoxus does not occur.

19. On the resting adult electrocardiogram T wave inversion

A in a VI is always abnormal
B in V_2 is always abnormal
C in V_5 is always abnormal
D may be seen in subendocardial ischaemia
E may be generalised in pericarditis

Your answers: A.........B.........C.........D.........E.........

20. The following statements are correct for the normal adult resting electrocardiogram:

A the mean frontal plane QRS axis is between 0° and +90°
B the mean frontal plane T wave axis may not differ from the mean frontal plane QRS axis by more than 45°
C the P wave should not exceed a height of 0.25 mV or duration of 0.12 seconds
D in the praecordial leads at least one R wave should exceed a height of 8 mm (0.8 mV) but no R wave should be greater than 27 mm (2.7 mV)
E the sum of the tallest R wave in the left praecordial leads and the deepest S wave in the right praecordial leads must not exceed 30 mm

Your answers: A.........B.........C.........D.........E.........

21. During normal inspiration

A right atrial pressure increases
B pulmonary venous flow increases
C systemic arterial pressure increases
D heart rate decreases
E splitting of the second heart sound is increased

Your answers: A.........B.........C.........D.........E.........

Answers overleaf

19. C D E

T wave inversion occurs in V_1 in 20% of normal adults and in V_2 in 5% of normal adults (who also have T wave inversion in V_1). T wave inversion in V_3 - V_6 and I and II is always abnormal in adults. T wave inversion may be normal in aVL, aVf and III, but only if the mean frontal plane T wave axis does not differ greatly from the mean frontal plane QRS axis. Abnormal T wave inversion can be due to ischaemia, strain or pericarditis.

20. B C D

The mean frontal plane QRS axis should lie between –30° and +90°. Left ventricular hypertrophy is present if the sum of the tallest R wave in the left praecordial leads and the deepest S wave in the right praecordial leads exceeds 40 mm. Left ventricular hypertrophy can also be diagnosed by the presence of a tall R wave (over 27 mm) in the left praecordial leads alone. Small amplitude R waves may be due to myxoedema or a pericardial effusion. Tall P waves suggest right atrial hypertrophy and broad P waves suggest left atrial hypertrophy.

21. E

During inspiration the intrathoracic pressure decreases, so that blood is drawn into the lung vessels. As a result blood is sucked through the right side of the heart into the lungs, but prevented from flowing out of the pulmonary veins into the systemic circulation. The right atrial and systemic arterial pressures decrease and heart rate increases. The increased blood flow through the right ventricle and decreased flow through the left ventricle means that pulmonary valve closure is delayed and aortic valve closure is earlier, which exaggerates the normal splitting of the second heart sound.

22. The following statements about the cardiac output are correct:

A in an adult of average size the cardiac output at rest is approximately 5 litres/minute

B in an adult of average size the total oxygen consumption at rest is about 5 litres/minute

C the Fick principle for measuring cardiac output requires a knowledge of oxygen consumption, heart rate and blood pressure

D the thermodilution methods of measuring cardiac output are affected by recirculation of the indicator

E cardiac output is increased by reducing the afterload on the heart

Your answers: A.........B.........C.........D.........E.........

23. Atrial myxomas

A are more common in the right atrium than in the left atrium

B do not recur after resection

C may mimic infective endocarditis

D are poorly visualised on echocardiography

E usually arise from a pedicle near to the fossa ovalis

Your answers: A.........B.........C.........D.........E.........

24. A broad complex tachycardia is more likely to be supraventricular tachycardia with aberrant conduction than ventricular tachycardia if

A cannon waves are seen in the neck veins

B fusion beats are seen on the electrocardiogram

C atrioventricular dissociation is seen on the electrocardiogram

D the QRS complexes are morphologically identical to a bundle branch block pattern seen when the patient is in sinus rhythm

E the tachycardia is abolished by carotid sinus massage

Your answers: A.........B.........C.........D.........E.........

Answers overleaf

22. A E

Determination of cardiac output by the Fick method requires a knowledge of the arteriovenous oxygen difference (i.e. systemic arterial – pulmonary arterial oxygen contents) and total oxygen consumption. In an adult of average size the resting oxygen consumption is about 250 ml/minute, which is derived from a respiratory minute volume of about 5 litres/minute. Thermodilution methods of measuring cardiac output are unaffected by recirculation since the small volume of cold saline injected is rapidly warmed during transit through the tissues. Recirculation is however a significant problem for dye dilution methods.

23. C E

Atrial myxomas usually arise near to the fossa ovalis. They are twice as common in the left atrium as in the right. They cause valve dysfunction, emboli, fever, joint pains, a raised ESR and anaemia. Thus the findings are often similar to those of infective endocarditis. The tumours are well visualised on echocardiography. After resection the tumour may recur particularly if any part of the pedicle is not removed.

24. D E

During ventricular tachycardia the atria continue their own independent activity, unless retrograde activation of the atria is occurring through the atrioventricular node. Evidence of atrial activity independent of the ventricular tachycardia include cannon waves (when atria and ventricles coincidentally contract simultaneously), atrioventricular dissociation and fusion beats on the ECG. Supraventricular tachycardia is quite often abolished by carotid sinus massage but ventricular tachycardia is not. When the pattern of ventricular activation during the tachycardia is the same as sometimes occurs during sinus rhythm, this strongly suggests the presence of supraventricular tachycardia with aberrant conduction.

25. In patients with bradycardia, atrioventricular dual chamber (sequential or DDD) pacing

A increases cardiac output compared with ventricular demand pacing
B improves survival compared with ventricular demand pacing
C is less likely to produce pacemaker mediated tachycardia than ventricular demand pacing
D increases exercise performance compared with ventricular demand pacing
E is the method of choice for physiological pacing of patients in atrial fibrillation

Your answers: A.........B.........C.........D.........E.........

26. Treatment with thiazide diuretics

A improves glucose tolerance
B reduces potassium loss
C may precipitate uraemia in patients with impaired renal function
D may precipitate gout
E reduces circulating renin levels

Your answers: A.........B.........C.........D.........E.........

27. The following statements are correct for aortic stenosis:

A syncope typically occurs on exertion
B angina means that coronary artery disease is also present
C unless treated surgically, development of symptoms is typically followed by rapid progression and death
D when aortic stenosis is severe reverse splitting of the second heart sound occurs
E pure aortic stenosis is usually rheumatic in origin

Your answers: A.........B.........C.........D.........E.........

Answers overleaf

25. A D

Dual chamber pacing is used either to sense or stimulate the atria followed, after an appropriate interval, by ventricular pacing. It is therefore physiological and improves haemodynamics compared with ventricular demand pacemaking. Cardiac output and exercise performance are improved but survival is not. Dual chamber pacing is more expensive and more complicated than ventricular demand pacing. Dual chamber pacing is also more likely to precipitate a pacemaker induced tachycardia, particularly if retrograde atrioventricular conduction is possible through the patient's bundle of His. Dual chamber pacing is ineffective in atrial fibrillation when other types of rate responsive pacemakers are used.

26. C D

Thiazides decrease sodium transport in the distal tubule just proximal to the site of potassium exchange. They increase potassium loss by delivery of more sodium to the distal tubule where potassium exchange occurs and by producing secondary hyperaldosteronism. Renin secretion is increased. If a large diuresis occurs dehydration and uraemia can be precipitated, particularly in those with impaired renal function. Thiazides also reduce urate excretion by the kidneys and can precipitate gout. Thiazides decrease carbohydrate tolerance, probably by reducing insulin secretion and can precipitate diabetes mellitus.

27. A C D

Pure aortic stenosis at a young age is usually the result of a congenitally abnormal valve and in later life due to calcification. Symptom development is an ominous sign. Typically symptoms occur on exertion, notably angina, dyspnoea, dizziness or syncope. Angina can occur despite normal coronary arteries because of the large myocardial oxygen demand. In severe aortic stenosis valve closure occurs late. It may be simultaneous with the pulmonary valve closure in inspiration and after the pulmonary valve closure in expiration when there is said to be reversed splitting. Sometimes, the aortic valve is so immobile that the aortic component of the second sound is inaudible.

28. The following statements are correct for infective endocarditis:

A infective endocarditis should be considered in all patients with a murmur and fever

B in the elderly, infective endocarditis characteristically presents with confusion and no fever

C persistent fever after more than one week of bactericidal concentrations of appropriate antibiotics is characteristically due to either allergy to the medication or extensive infection requiring surgical treatment.

D infective endocarditis should be considered in drug addicts with pleurisy

E infective endocarditis occurring soon after cardiac surgery is characteristically due to Streptococci of the viridans type

Your answers: A.........B.........C.........D.........E.........

29. During pregnancy

A cardiac output increases

B a cardiomyopathy may occur

C new cardiac murmurs are usually innocent

D use of anticoagulants is a more difficult problem than in non-pregnant women

E pulmonary oedema due to mitral stenosis is characteristically treated by valvotomy

Your answers: A.........B.........C.........D.........E.........

30. The following statements are correct for mitral regurgitation:

A the severity of mitral regurgitation is improved by reducing left ventricular afterload

B in severe mitral regurgitation with a giant left atrium, a large v wave is characteristically observed in the left atrial pressure trace

C the first heart sound is characteristically loud

D mitral regurgitation is an important cause of acute cardiac failure following myocardial infarction

E a murmur confined to late systole suggests subvalvar mitral regurgitation

Your answers: A.........B.........C.........D.........E.........

Answers overleaf

28. A B C D

Infective endocarditis should be considered in all patients with fever and a murmur. However, fever may be absent in the elderly, those immunosuppressed or on steroids. A murmur is not always heard, especially when right heart endocarditis is present. Right heart endocarditis is likely to occur in those who abuse intravenous drugs because of use of infected needles. Right heart endocarditis typically produces infected pulmonary emboli. Infective endocarditis following cardiac surgery is usually due to staphylococci or fungi acquired during the operation.

29. A B C D E

During pregnancy cardiac output increases and new murmurs are usually innocent flow murmurs. However, a cardiomyopathy is well described in association with pregnancy and pre-existing cardiac lesions are more likely to present at this time of increased cardiac work. Mitral stenosis requiring surgery during pregnancy is usually treated by valvotomy. Use of anticoagulants in pregnant women (or young women who may subsequently become pregnant) does present problems. Oral anticoagulants are teratogenic and can cross the placenta with the risk of placental and fetal haemorrhage.

30. A D E

Mitral regurgitation produces a dominant v wave on the left atrial pressure trace. However, if the left atrium is very large the compliance of the chamber will prevent a large amplitude wave being observed. Characteristically the first heart sound is soft and a pan-systolic murmur is heard, but in subvalvar mitral regurgitation a late systolic murmur is characteristic. Papillary muscle dysfunction after myocardial infarction may precipitate mitral regurgitation and acute pulmonary oedema. Reducing left ventricular afterload increases forward flow and reduces mitral regurgitation.

31. In a patient with rheumatic mitral valve disease, sudden onset of severe dyspnoea and an increase in the systolic murmur is typically due to

A pulmonary embolism
B myocardial infarction
C rupture of chordae tendinae
D infective endocarditis
E onset of atrial fibrillation

Your answers: A.........B.........C.........D.........E.........

32. The following statements are correct for mitral valve leaflet prolapse:

A the milder forms of this condition may be considered a normal variant
B the valve is regurgitant if a mitral systolic murmur is present in addition to a mid-systolic click
C antibiotic prophylaxis for dental and surgical treatment is unnecessary because there is no increase in the risk of infective endocarditis
D the murmur becomes quieter when phenylephrine is given
E mitral leaflet prolapse is associated with systemic embolisation

Your answers: A.........B.........C.........D.........E.........

33. In a patient with aortic regurgitation and fever the following are very ominous prognostic signs when associated with onset of severe breathlessness:

A absent first heart sound
B increase in length and loudness of the aortic diastolic murmur
C increase in pulse pressure
D a pericardial rub
E onset of complete heart block

Your answers: A.........B.........C.........D.........E.........

Answers overleaf

31. C D

In a patient with rheumatic mitral valve disease, any of the above conditions could produce a sudden onset of severe dyspnoea but only rupture of chordae tendinae and infective endocarditis characteristically increase the systolic murmu by increasing the amount of valvular regurgitation. Atria fibrillation and pulmonary embolism are recognised feature of rheumatic heart disease and myocardial infarction ca result from coronary embolism. The chordae tendinae of mitra valves are damaged by the rheumatic process and rupture i well recognised.

32. A E

Mitral leaflet prolapse varies from gross and pathological t mild when it is a normal variant occurring in about 10% of th population. In the gross cases complications are a real risk These include systemic embolisation, cardiac dysrhythmia and infective endocarditis. Antibiotic prophylaxis is recom mended for all but the most mild cases, when the risk c anaphylaxis due to the antibiotics probably exceeds the risk c endocarditis. A good clinical guide is to give prophylaxis t those who have a murmur but not to those with only a click. murmur does not necessarily mean mitral regurgitation i present. Anything which increases left ventricular size (e.g phenylephrine) will make the murmur louder.

33. A D E

In a patient with fever and aortic regurgitation the most impo tant diagnosis to be considered is infective endocarditis. In thi setting, severe worsening of the aortic regurgitation is ind cated by absence or softness of the first heart sound (due t premature closure of the mitral valve), reduction of puls pressure and shortening of the diastolic murmur becaus these suggest that there is almost free aortic regurgitation an a high left ventricular end-diastolic pressure. A pericardial ru and the onset of complete heart block suggest extension of th infective process into the pericardium or myocardium respec tively.

34. The following statements are correct for aortic regurgitation:

- A in a child, severe aortic regurgitation is most frequently associated with an atrial septal defect
- B the presence of an aortic ejection systolic murmur is due to associated aortic stenosis
- C the onset of heart failure requires urgent investigation with a view to valve replacement
- D angina suggests the possibility of syphilitic aortitis
- E good blood pressure control typically abolishes aortic regurgitation due to hypertension

Your answers: A.........B.........C.........D.........E.........

35. Following a myocardial infarction the following are adverse prognostic factors:

- A young age
- B inferior transmural infarction
- C right bundle branch block
- D hypertension
- E first myocardial infarction

Your answers: A.........B.........C.........D.........E.........

36. The following statements are correct of beta-blockers:

- A beta-blockers reduce blood pressure by vasodilatation
- B beta-blockers control the symptoms of thyrotoxicosis
- C beta-blockers are used alone to treat hypertension due to a phaeochromocytoma
- D beta-blockers may mask the symptoms of hypoglycaemia
- E beta-blockers reduce angina by dilating the coronary arteries

Your answers: A.........B.........C.........D.........E.........

Answers overleaf

34. C D E

In patients with aortic regurgitation a systolic murmur characteristically occurs due to the high systolic flow without significant valve narrowing. In children aortic regurgitation is usually associated with a ventricular septal defect. In adults aortic regurgitation in a patient with angina should prompt investigations to exclude syphilitic aortitis, although coincidental coronary artery disease is common. Aortic regurgitation due to hypertension may be abolished purely by adequate blood pressure control. However, in those with symptomatic aortic regurgitation, cardiac catheterisation is indicated.

35. None of the answers is correct

Following a myocardial infarction the adverse prognostic factors are advanced age, anterior transmural infarction, history of previous myocardial infarction, left bundle branch block, heart failure, hypotension and complex ventricular arrhythmias occurring late after the infarction. Most of these adverse prognostic factors are indicators of extensive myocardial damage.

36. B D

Beta-blockers reduce the rate and force of contraction of the heart. They reduce angina and blood pressure by reducing the amount of cardiac work done. They are vasoconstrictors. They should not be used alone to treat a phaeochromocytoma, which secretes noradrenaline (alpha stimulant) and adrenaline (alpha and beta stimulant). The hypertension of phaeochromocytomas is therefore controlled with predominantly alpha blocking agents and beta-blockers have a secondary role. If beta-blockers are used alone to treat a phaeochromocytoma blood pressure may rise further. An alternative is to block synthesis of the neurotransmitters with alpha-methyl-tyrosine which is converted to a false transmitter, and then surgically remove the tumour.

37. The following measures have been shown to improve survival after a myocardial infarction:

A early thrombolytic therapy
B therapy with a calcium antagonist
C therapy with intravenous nitrates
D training of the general public in basic life support (cardio-pulmonary resuscitation)
E therapy with beta-blockers

Your answers: A.........B.........C.........D.........E.........

38. The following statements are correct for electromechanical dissociation:

A the electrocardiogram shows no cardiac activity
B it responds to DC cardioversion
C it has a better prognosis than ventricular fibrillation
D electromechanical dissociation occurring a week after acute myocardial infarction is characteristically the result of cardiac rupture.
E it may respond to adrenaline injected down an endotracheal tube if intravenous access is not available

Your answers: A.........B.........C.........D.........E.........

39. The following statements are correct for heart block:

A the Wenckebach phenomenon may occur in healthy individuals
B after an acute anterior myocardial infarction, development of bifascicular block has a poor prognosis
C in asymptomatic individuals, the chance finding of slight lengthening of the PR interval is of no significance
D patients with recurrent symptomatic episodes of complete heart block should be given a trial of oral isoprenaline before consideration for permanent pacemaker implantation
E complete heart block developing during the first day after an inferior myocardial infarction will usually require permanent pacing because the artery to the atrioventricular node is involved in the disease territory

Your answers: A.........B.........C.........D.........E.........

Answers overleaf

37. A D E

Adequate training of the general public in basic life support is a highly effective method of reducing early arrhythmic deaths following acute myocardial infarction. There is increasing evidence that thrombolytic therapy if administered in the first few hours and treatment with beta- blockers improve prognosis of myocardial infarction. There is no evidence that calcium antagonists or nitrates improve prognosis.

38. D E

Electromechanical dissociation causes cardiac arrest. The ECG shows complexes but there is no mechanical activity or pulse. It has a worse prognosis than either ventricular fibrillation or asystole. It may be due to cardiac rupture. Other causes are cardiac depressant drugs, tension pneumothorax and cardiac tamponade. It is treated with drugs, particularly adrenaline, but also isoprenaline and calcium. Adrenaline may be injected down the trachea and will be absorbed into the pulmonary veins and so reach the heart if effective external cardiac massage is being performed.

39. A B C

First degree heart block and the Wenckebach phenomenon occur in healthy individuals. Bifascicular block after an acute anterior myocardial infarction is associated with a mortality of about 50% since it means a large amount of cardiac tissue has been damaged. Complete heart block may occur with inferior myocardial infarction since the artery to the atrioventricular node arises from the right coronary artery, but the heart block usually resolves in a few days without requiring permanent pacing. Oral isoprenaline should not be used as first line therapy to treat episodes of complete heart block. It may precipitate ventricular arrhythmias and permanent pacing is preferable.

40. The following statements are correct for myocardial infarction (MI):

A few people who have ECG evidence of MI give no history of chest pain compatible with such a diagnosis
B a significant proportion of patients who have myocardial infarction have no history of angina
C in the hours after a myocardial infarction the probability of ventricular fibrillation increases progressively
D new Q waves signify a recent transmural MI
E presence of old, deep Q waves always signifies a previous transmural myocardial infarction, except in lead aVr

Your answers: A.........B.........C.........D.........E.........

41. The following statements are correct for hypertension:

A life expectancy is improved by reducing the blood pressure in all groups of patients whose arterial diastolic pressure exceeds 90 mm Hg
B the presence of hypertension and hyperkalaemia suggests Conn's syndrome
C the presence of hypertension, obesity and hyperkalaemia suggests Cushing's syndrome
D after repair of a coarctation of the aorta the blood pressure often remains elevated unless treated medically
E phaeochromocytomas may occur outside the adrenals

Your answers: A.........B.........C.........D.........E.........

42. The following statements are correct for pulmonary embolism (PE):

A a clinical picture similar to primary pulmonary hypertension is recognised as resulting from recurrent small PE
B measurement of arterial gases whilst breathing air after PE typically shows a raised PCO_2 and reduced PO_2
C after pulmonary embolism, the right atrial pressure may exceed left atrial pressure
D PE typically originate from leg or pelvic venous thrombi
E demonstration of the presence of PE by ventilation/perfusion lung scanning is easy and entirely safe

Your answers: A.........B.........C.........D.........E.........

Answers overleaf

40. B D

30-40% of people who have myocardial infarctions have no angina and one quarter of those with ECG evidence of old infarction give no history of severe chest pain or other symptoms in keeping with such a diagnosis. Development of new Q waves on the ECG signifies recent infarction, but Q waves can be present on the ECG without infarction. Q waves can occur in the presence of normal coronary arteries in cardiomyopathies, lung disease and left bundle branch block. Q waves are normal in aVr. After a myocardial infarction, the probability of developing ventricular fibrillation is maximal early and decreases progressively.

41. D E

There is no evidence that the prognosis of mildly hypertensive patients is improved by treatment. Because of the raised circulating levels of adrenocortical steroids in Conn's and Cushing's syndromes there is a tendency for hypokalaemia. After repair of coarctation of the aorta, most patients still require antihypertensive medication. 10% of phaeochromocytomas occur outside the adrenals in other sympathetic ganglia; 10% are bilateral and 10% are malignant.

42. A C D

Pulmonary emboli usually originate from thrombi in the lower limbs and pelvis. When recurrent, they may produce pulmonary hypertension and right heart failure. However, more characteristically there are single episodes of dyspnoea, chest pain and haemoptysis, at which time arterial gases show a reduced PO_2 and reduced PCO_2. The jugular venous pressure is often raised and right atrial pressure may exceed left atrial pressure. Pulmonary emboli can be demonstrated by lung scanning or angiography, but neither technique is entirely free from risk of sudden deterioration and death of the patient.

43. The following statements are correct for cardiac failure:

A cardiac failure is due to dilated cardiomyopathy if the heart chambers are enlarged and the coronary arteries and cardiac valves are normal

B cardiac failure is usually treated with diuretics, since these improve breathlessness on exertion and reduce oedema

C angiotensin converting enzyme inhibitors improve exercise performance and life expectancy in patients with cardiac failure

D serious arrhythmias and sudden death are a major cause of mortality in patients with cardiac failure, whether or not they have normal coronary arteries

E oedema occurs when the oncotic pressure of the plasma proteins exceeds the hydrostatic pressure across the capillary wall

Your answers: A.........B.........C.........D.........E.........

44. Cannon waves may be observed in the jugular veins in

A constrictive pericarditis

B first degree heart block

C tricuspid stenosis

D ventricular pacing

E nodal tachycardia

Your answers: A.........B.........C.........D.........E.........

45. In patients with accessory atrioventricular pathways the resting electrocardiogram commonly

A shows a prolonged PR interval

B shows a prolonged QT interval

C shows a delta wave

D appears normal

E shows complete heart block

Your answers: A.........B.........C.........D.........E.........

Answers overleaf

43. A B C D

Oedema occurs when the hydrostatic pressure across the capillary wall exceeds the plasma protein oncotic pressure. Although there are a number of agents which improve symptoms in patients with heart failure, there has been little impact on the long-term mortality, with many patients dying suddenly and from arrhythmias, rather than progressive heart failure.

44. D E

Cannon waves occur when the atria contract against closed atrioventricular valves, i.e. during ventricular systole. They occur irregularly during complete heart block and ventricular pacing when the atrial rate is independent of the ventricular rate. Cannon waves can also occur regularly during nodal tachycardia if retrograde activation of the atria occurs synchronously with ventricular contraction. In tricuspid stenosis there is a dominant a wave and in constrictive pericarditis the jugular venous pressure trace shows a dominant y descent. The venous pressure trace appears normal in first degree heart block.

45. C D

In patients with accessory atrioventricular pathways premature excitation of the ventricles occurs via congenital anomalous conduction pathways which result in a short PR interval. A delta wave may be present (Wolff-Parkinson-White syndrome) or absent (Lown-Ganong-Levine syndrome). The QRS complex may be otherwise normal or may resemble bundle branch block depending on the pattern of activation of the ventricles. On occasions conduction through the accessory pathway is blocked, so that the ECG appears normal.

46. Atrial fibrillation is a characteristic presenting feature of

A alcoholic cardiomyopathy
B thyrotoxicosis
C diphtheritic cardiomyopathy
D Reiter's syndrome
E rheumatic fever

Your answers: A.........B.........C.........D.........E.........

47. Major criteria of rheumatic fever include

A prolonged PR interval
B arthralgia
C chorea
D erythema nodosum
E subcutaneous nodules

Your answers: A.........B.........C.........D.........E.........

48. In hypertrophic obstructive cardiomyopathy

A the pulse is slow rising
B an atrial impulse is characteristically detected
C the systolic murmur characteristically decreases on squatting
D an aortic diastolic murmur is a recognised feature
E echocardiography is usually unhelpful

Your answers: A.........B.........C.........D.........E.........

Answers overleaf

46. A B

Atrial fibrillation is common in patients with ischaemic heart disease, cor pulmonale, thyrotoxicosis, many types of cardiomyopathies and rheumatic heart disease. It is not common in acute rheumatic fever, Reiter's syndrome or diphtheritic cardiomyopathy when conduction problems are more frequent.

47. C E

Rheumatic fever is diagnosed by the presence of two major criteria or one major and two minor criteria in a patient with a history of a recent streptococcal infection. Major criteria of rheumatic fever are carditis, polyarthritis, chorea, erythema marginatum and subcutaneous nodules. Minor criteria are a history of rheumatic fever, arthralgia, fever, raised ESR, raised C reactive protein, leucocytosis and first degree heart block.

48. B C

In hypertrophic obstructive cardiomyopathy the pulse is characteristically jerky and an atrial impulse is detected. The systolic murmur is decreased by squatting and isometric exercise which increase the left ventricular cavity size, but manoeuvres which reduce the cavity size (Valsalva manoeuvre and standing) increase the murmur. Unlike aortic valve disease and discrete subvalvar stenosis, aortic regurgitation is not a feature of hypertrophic cardiomyopathy. The diagnosis is usually confirmed by echocardiography.

49. The following statements are correct for mitral stenosis:

A the later the opening snap the more severe the stenosis
B mitral stenosis is approximately equally common in men and women
C a loud first heart sound suggests a rigid or calcified valve
D presystolic accentuation of the diastolic murmur occurs if the patient is in atrial fibrillation
E the Graham Steell murmur is due to associated aortic incompetence

Your answers: A.........B.........C.........D.........E.........

50. The following measures are used in the treatment of severe left ventricular failure:

A disopyramide infusion
B noradrenaline infusion
C nitroprusside infusion
D dobutamine infusion
E mechanical ventilation

Your answers: A.........B.........C.........D.........E.........

Answers overleaf

49. None of the answers is correct

The first sound and the opening snap become softer as the valve calcifies and becomes rigid. The opening snap gets earlier as the disease progresses because the left atrial pressure rises and thus exceeds left ventricular pressure earlier in diastole. Presystolic accentuation of the diastolic murmur is due to atrial contraction, so it disappears with the onset of atrial fibrillation. The early diastolic murmur described by Graham Steell is due to pulmonary regurgitation. Mitral stenosis is 3-4 times more common in women than men.

50. C D E

Left ventricular failure can be treated by reducing the preload and afterload on the left ventricle (e.g. vasodilators like nitroprusside, diuretics and sedatives) or with positive inotropic agents which also possess vasodilator properties (e.g. dobutamine). Noradrenaline has little inotropic action and has a powerful vasoconstrictor effect, it generally makes heart failure worse by increasing preload and afterload. Mechanical ventilation can be used to relieve patients of the work of respiration and positive end expiratory pressure ventilation (PEEP) helps to reduce pulmonary oedema by increasing alveolar pressure. Antiarrhythmic drugs are generally negatively inotropic and should be avoided unless specifically indicated.

Indicate your answers by putting T (True), F (False) or D (Don't know) in the spaces provided.

51. Asbestosis

A may be diagnosed by finding asbestos bodies in the sputum
B produces a restrictive lung defect
C is usually unresponsive to treatment with corticosteroids
D usually progresses even after exposure to asbestos has ceased
E is associated with finger clubbing

Your answers: A.........B.........C.........D.........E.........

52. The following organisms may cause a lobar pneumonia in previously healthy individuals with normal lungs:

A *Staphylococcus aureus*
B *Mycoplasma pneumoniae*
C *Haemophilus influenzae*
D *Legionella pneumophila*
E *Mycobacterium tuberculosis*

Your answers: A.........B.........C.........D.........E.........

53. The following statements are correct:

A pulmonary blood flow is greatest at the lung apices
B the carotid sinus is a chemoreceptor, monitoring arterial PO_2 and PCO_2
C in normal individuals, respiration is stimulated when arterial PO_2 falls below about 85 mm Hg (11.3 kPa)
D mean pulmonary artery pressure in normals is about 30 mm Hg (4 kPa)
E in normals, the total resistance in the pulmonary circulation is about half that in the systemic circulation

Your answers: A.........B.........C.........D.........E.........

Answers overleaf

51. B C D E

Asbestos bodies in the sputum merely indicate past exposure to asbestos, not necessarily asbestosis. It is important to differentiate between asbestosis (pulmonary fibrosis caused by asbestos fibres in the lung) and other pulmonary problems caused by asbestos, mainly benign pleural disease and malignant mesothelioma. As with other causes of pulmonary fibrosis, a restrictive picture and finger clubbing are usual. Asbestos fibres may remain in the lung for decades so progression occurs even without further asbestos exposure.

52. A B D E

Staph. aureus pneumonia is particularly common during influenza epidemics. Diagnosis of *Mycoplasma pneumonia* may be suggested by the presence of cold agglutinins, reportedly found in 30-75% of cases. *H. influenzae* characteristically causes infection in subjects with pre-existing bronchitis or bronchiectasis. *L. pneumophila* may be acquired from air conditioning systems and showers in hotels and hospitals. *M. tuberculosis* may cause a surprisingly acute lobar pneumonia.

53. All false

Mean pulmonary artery pressure in normal man is about 15 mm Hg (2 kPa). The effects of gravity therefore mean that the apices of the lungs are barely perfused at all in the upright position. Resistance to pulmonary blood flow is about 10% of that in the systemic circulation. The carotid sinus is primarily a baroreceptor, the adjacent carotid body being the peripheral arterial chemoreceptor. Hypoxic stimulation of respiration occurs when PaO_2 is below about 65 mm Hg (8.7 kPa); usually, any tendency to rise in $PaCO_2$ stimulates respiration before accompanying hypoxia does.

54. The following drugs may result in pulmonary fibrosis:

A busulphan
B bleomycin
C methotrexate
D amiodarone
E erythromycin

Your answers: A.........B.........C.........D.........E.........

55. The following may cause extrinsic allergic alveolitis:

A colophony resin used in soldering flux
B avian serum protein and droppings
C *Micropolyspora* and *Thermoactinomyces* species present in mouldy hay
D platinum salts
E cat fur

Your answers: A.........B.........C.........D.........E.........

56. In small cell anaplastic carcinoma of the bronchus (oat cell carcinoma)

A median survival from time of diagnosis is about 14 months in untreated patients
B metastases are usually present at the time of diagnosis
C chemotherapy is the initial treatment of choice
D the tumour is usually resistant to treatment with radio-therapy
E inappropriate antidiuretic hormone secretion is a recognised association

Your answers: A.........B.........C.........D.........E.........

Answers overleaf

54. A B C D

Drugs A – D may result in diffuse lung disease which can closely resemble cryptogenic fibrosing alveolitis. Other drugs with similar effects include nitrofurantoin and hexamethonium (formerly used to treat hypertension). Ingestion of the weedkiller paraquat produces an acute and progressive, usually rapidly fatal fibrosis.

55. B C

The antigens in B and C cause the conditions commonly known as bird fanciers' lung and farmers' lung respectively. Mediated by a Type III hypersensitivity reaction, and associated with precipitating antibodies, this is a mainly alveolar reaction to inhalation of these organic dusts. Acute attacks are associated with cough, dyspnoea, fever, malaise and hypoxia. With chronic exposure irreversible pulmonary fibrosis may result. Antigens in A and D are responsible for occupational asthma, mediated by Type I hypersensitivity.

56. B C E

Small cell anaplastic carcinoma of the bronchus is a rapidly growing tumour, the median survival from time of diagnosis being about 3-4 months in untreated patients. Although the tumour is usually radiosensitive, widespread metastatic disease is almost invariably present at the time of diagnosis so systemic chemotherapy with cytotoxic drugs is the treatment of choice. Radiotherapy may be used for the palliation of troublesome individual bony or cerebral metastases. Surgery is only considered after exhaustive search for spread of disease; even so, most of the very small number surgically treated die from previously undetected metastases.

57. In emphysema

A airways resistance is increased
B total lung capacity is reduced
C carbon monoxide transfer factor is normal or raised
D functional residual capacity is increased
E static lung compliance is increased

Your answers: A.........B.........C.........D.........E.........

58. Radiological pulmonary shadowing and a blood eosinophilia may be associated with

A extrinsic allergic alveolitis
B *Ascaris lumbricoides*
C aspirin
D *Aspergillus fumigatus*
E polyarteritis nodosa

Your answers: A.........B.........C.........D.........E.........

59. In miliary tuberculosis

A the chest radiograph may be normal
B a negative tuberculin test excludes the diagnosis
C there may be associated hypokalaemia
D patients may have no symptoms or signs other than mild pyrexia
E tuberculous meningitis is uncommon

Your answers: A.........B.........C.........D.........E.........

Answers overleaf

57. A D E

Emphysema is dilatation and destruction of airspaces distal to the terminal bronchioles; gas transfer is reduced. Loss of elastic recoil increases the tendency to airways collapse during expiration; air trapping occurs distal to closed airways and subjects breathe at higher lung volumes to minimise airways collapse. With loss of elastic recoil lung distension (change in lung volume with change in intrapleural pressure) is easier so compliance is increased when measured by the static method.

58. B C D E

Extrinsic allergic alveolitis, largely due to Type III hypersensitivity with precipitating antibodies in the serum is characteristically not associated with eosinophilia. *Ascaris lumbricoides, Ancylostomum braziliense* and *Trichuris trichiura* are the commonest parasites associated with pulmonary shadows and eosinophilia. Aspirin, para-amino salicylic acid, phenylbutazone, nitrofurantoin and methotrexate may also be responsible. *Aspergillus fumigatus* is the commonest cause of so-called asthmatic pulmonary eosinophilia in Great Britain. Lung involvement and eosinophilia are present in about one third of cases of polyarteritis nodosa.

59. A C D

Miliary tuberculosis results from haematogenous dissemination of tubercle bacilli. The classic radiographic picture of multiple "millet seed" size pulmonary lesions, a few mm in diameter, gives the condition its name but the chest X-ray may be normal for months before development of miliary shadows. Patients, particularly the elderly, may be mildly unwell with only unexplained anaemia or fever for long periods before diagnosis. The tuberculin test may be negative, particularly in the very ill. Hypokalaemia is well recognised but poorly understood. Up to 50% of children with miliary tuberculosis have tuberculous meningitis at the time of presentation.

60. Infection with the following viruses may result in pneumonia:

A measles
B mumps
C varicella
D rubella
E cytomegalovirus

Your answers: A.........B.........C.........D.........E.........

61. In childhood asthma

A the only symptom may be nocturnal cough
B a single dose of inhaled cromoglycate will often prevent exercise induced asthma
C house dust mite allergy is common
D inhaled steroids may lead to growth retardation and Cushing's syndrome
E peak expiratory flow rates are generally at their lowest values at the end of the day

Your answers: A.........B.........C.........D.........E.........

62. The following conditions may involve the lung:

A Wegener's granulomatosis
B haemochromatosis
C syphilis
D leptospirosis
E gout

Your answers: A.........B.........C.........D.........E.........

Answers overleaf

60. A C E

Bacterial pneumonia may complicate measles infection but the virus itself may be responsible for bronchopneumonia or a miliary radiographic picture. Varicella (chickenpox) pneumonia is relatively commoner in adults, affecting up to about one third of adult cases of chickenpox. The illness is often severe. Nodular radiographic shadows may later go on to calcify, resulting in a striking picture of miliary calcification. Cytomegalovirus infection is commonly subclinical, but in other individuals pneumonia may be present along with the other clinical features resembling infectious mononucleosis. In immunosuppressed individuals and the newborn, infection may be very severe and even fatal.

61. A B C

Cough may be the only symptom of hyper-reactive airways and, like other symptoms of asthma, is usually worse at night and early in the morning. Cromoglycate will not treat an asthmatic attack once started and generally must be used regularly as prophylaxis, but is surprisingly effective taken immediately before exercise. In conventional dosage, the only side effects attributable to inhaled steroids are an increased tendency to oral thrush *(Candida)* and occasionally, hoarseness of the voice.

62. A C D

In classical Wegener's granulomatosis there is glomerulonephritis, generalised vasculitis and necrotising granulomata in the respiratory tract. As originally described, the lesions were in the upper respiratory tract, but pulmonary manifestations are common. Secondary syphilis may cause cough and sputum, with a bronchopneumonic clinical and radiological picture. Pulmonary involvement is frequent in leptospirosis, with cough and sputum, and patchy or confluent infiltrates visible radiologically.

63. Hilar lymphadenopathy is a recognised feature of

A aspergilloma
B streptococcal pneumonia
C sarcoidosis
D pulmonary involvement by rheumatoid disease
E tuberculosis

Your answers: A.........B.........C.........D.........E.........

64. Erythromycin is appropriate treatment for pulmonary infections with the following organisms:

A *Legionella pneumophila*
B *Pneumocystis carinii*
C *Cryptococcus neoformans*
D *Pseudomonas aeruginosa*
E *Mycoplasma pneumoniae*

Your answers: A.........B.........C.........D.........E.........

65. The following may be used in the treatment of asthma:

A pirbuterol
B acebutolol
C rimiterol
D ipratropium
E budesonide

Your answers: A.........B.........C.........D.........E.........

Answers overleaf

63. C E

In Great Britain, sarcoidosis is the commonest cause of bilateral hilar lymphadenopathy in patients over the age of 15 years. Unilateral enlargement occurs in only about 10% of cases of sarcoidosis. Such unilateral enlargement is suggestive of tuberculosis if present in a child, or neoplasm in an adult. Leukaemias (particularly lymphatic and lymphoblastic) and lymphomas must not be forgotten as causes of both unilateral and bilateral hilar enlargement, although the glands involved are more commonly mediastinal rather than hilar glands themselves.

64. A E

Erythromycin is probably the most effective antibiotic for *Legionella* and *Mycoplasma* infections, and for chlamydial and rickettsial lung infections. Tetracyclines and rifampicin are also sometimes used. The protozoan *Pneumocystis carinii* is usually treated with high dose co- trimoxazole or pentamidine. *Cryptococcus* requires antifungal agents like amphotericin *B. pseudomonas* is usually treated with two drugs, most often an aminoglycoside like gentamicin and a penicillin derivative like azlocillin or ticarcillin.

65. A C D E

Pirbuterol and rimiterol are ß-agonists. Other drugs in this group include salbutamol, terbutaline, fenoterol and reproterol. Acebutolol is a ß-blocker and is **contraindicated**. Ipratropium is an atropine-like parasympathetic blocker. Budesonide is a corticosteroid given by inhalation; other drugs in this group include beclomethasone and betamethasone.

66. A reduced carbon monoxide transfer factor is typically found in

A pulmonary haemorrhage
B an asthmatic between attacks
C left ventricular failure
D emphysema
E extrinsic allergic alveolitis

Your answers: A.........B.........C.........D.........E.........

67. Exposure to the following is associated with an increased risk of carcinoma of the bronchus:

A asbestos
B silica dust
C sulphur dioxide
D aniline dyes
E radon gas

Your answers: A.........B.........C.........D.........E.........

68. Arterial PO_2 may be reduced in acute overdose of

A benzodiazepines
B amitriptyline
C salicylates
D barbiturates
E paracetamol

Your answers: A.........B.........C.........D.........E.........

Answers overleaf

66. C D E

Carbon monoxide (CO) transfer factor measures gas transfer between alveoli and blood. Usually, a single breath of gas containing a known low concentration of CO is taken, held for 10 seconds, then expired. Measurement of expired gas volume and CO concentration enables calculation of CO uptake by blood flowing through pulmonary capillaries. When free blood is present in the bronchial tree, transfer factor is high as the haemoglobin binds the CO. Gas transfer is normal in asthmatics, but reduced in patients with emphysema due to destruction of gas exchanging surface and mismatching of ventilation and perfusion. A normal transfer factor in a 'bronchitic' or 'emphysematous' patient should always raise the possibility of asthma.

67. A E

Asbestos exposure increases the risk of developing carcinoma of the bronchus in smokers and non-smokers. Contrary to earlier teaching, asbestos may lead to bronchial carcinoma even when there is no asbestosis (i.e. pulmonary fibrosis due to asbestos fibres) present. Exposure to radon gas in miners was the first cause of occupational lung cancer to be described. There is no convincing evidence linking silica dust or sulphur dioxide with increased risk of bronchial carcinoma. Compounds formed during the manufacture of aniline dyes (but not the aniline dyes themselves) are associated with bladder cancer.

68. A B D

A, B and D all depress respiration in overdosage, with a fall in arterial PO_2 and rise in PCO_2; benzodiazepines generally cause less respiratory depression than other groups of sedative drugs. The arrhythmogenic effects of tricyclic antidepressants like amitriptyline are so well known that their capacity for profound respiratory depression is often forgotten. Paracetamol overdosage causes liver damage but not unconsciousness until hepatic failure has occurred. Salicylates directly stimulate the respiratory centre: arterial PO_2 is normal or high and a respiratory alkalosis is present. A patient with salicylate or paracetamol overdose who has respiratory depression with hypoxia has taken other drugs, usually dextropropoxyphene in the case of paracetamol.

69. The following are recognised features of pulmonary involvement by sarcoidosis:

A obstructive ventilatory defect
B inspiratory crackles heard on auscultation
C finger clubbing
D pleural effusion
E hypercalcaemia

Your answers: A.........B.........C.........D.........E.........

70. In carcinoma of the bronchus, the following suggest an inoperable lesion:

A a paralysed hemidiaphragm
B vocal cord palsy
C pleural effusion
D hypertrophic pulmonary osteoarthropathy
E peripheral neuropathy

Your answers: A.........B.........C.........D.........E.........

71. Cystic fibrosis

A is inherited as a sex-linked recessive trait
B is usually fatal by early teenage life
C *Klebsiella* is a common pulmonary pathogen
D sodium content of the sweat is increased
E male sufferers are infertile

Your answers: A.........B.........C.........D.........E.........

Answers overleaf

69. D E

A restrictive defect is the usual pattern of ventilatory impairment found in sarcoidosis; when disease is confined to hilar lymphadenopathy, or parenchymal involvement is minimal, spirometry may be normal. Inspiratory crackles and finger clubbing are not features of pulmonary sarcoidosis. Pleural effusions are uncommon but well described. Hypercalcaemia is due to (poorly understood) abnormalities of vitamin D metabolism; it may be particularly troublesome in those who work outdoors or patients who holiday in the sun.

70. A B C

A paralysed hemidiaphragm and vocal cord palsy suggest mediastinal involvement by tumour with damage to phrenic and recurrent laryngeal nerves respectively. In theory an effusion may be secondary to a pneumonia distal to an occluding but operable carcinoma. In practice it almost invariably implies pleural involvement by tumour or blockage of lymphatic drainage by tumour in mediastinal glands. D and E are non-metastatic manifestations of malignant disease, and may regress with removal of the tumour.

71. D E

Cystic fibrosis is inherited in an autosomal recessive fashion, and occurs in about 1 in 2000 live births in Great Britain. Over 50% of patients reach the age of 16 years and survival into the 30's and even 40's is becoming increasingly common. *Staphylococcus aureus* as the main pulmonary pathogen is usually replaced by *Pseudomonas aeruginosa* during adolescence. A cell membrane abnormality may be the underlying defect, one consequence of which is high sodium and chloride content in the sweat. Men are infertile; women have decreased fertility but may conceive.

72. The following are recognised associations of carcinoma of the bronchus:

A acanthosis nigricans
B dermatomyositis
C hyperkeratosis of palms and soles of feet
D cerebellar degeneration
E Cushing's syndrome

Your answers: A.........B.........C.........D.........E.........

73. In the normal postero-anterior chest radiograph

A the left lobe of the diaphragm is usually higher than the right
B the hilar shadows are principally composed of lymphoid tissue
C the right hilum is higher than the left
D loss of clarity of the left heart border suggests pathology in the lower lobe
E the lower trachea is deviated to the right

Your answers: A.........B.........C.........D.........E.........

74. The following statements are correct:

A the volume of air expired each minute is usually less than the volume inspired
B when arterial PO_2 is 70 mm Hg (9.3 kPa) the blood contains about 30% less oxygen than when PO_2 is 100 mm Hg (13.0 kPa)
C alveolar PO_2 is always greater than arterial PO_2
D a shift to the right of the oxygen dissociation curve implies a fall in the oxygen affinity of haemoglobin
E acidosis shifts the oxygen dissociation curve to the right

Your answers: A.........B.........C.........D.........E.........

Answers overleaf

72. A B D E

Acanthosis nigricans affects mucocutaneous junctions like the lips as well as the axillae and groin. The association between dermatomyositis and malignancy is less strong than was once thought, but probably about 10% of patients over 40 years of age have a tumour. Hyperkeratosis of soles and feet (tylosis) is a rare familial disorder associated with carcinoma of the oesophagus. Bronchial and ovarian carcinomas are the commonest tumours to cause cerebellar degeneration. Bronchial carcinomas, particularly small cell anaplastic (oat cell) tumours may secrete ACTH or peptides containing the ACTH sequence and so produce Cushing's syndrome.

73. E

In over 90% of normal subjects the right dome of the diaphragm is higher than the left; if much gas is present in the stomach they may temporarily be at the same level. Hilar shadows are composed of the pulmonary vessels, and to a small extent the walls of the major bronchi. The centre of the right hilum is roughly opposite the 3rd rib anteriorly; the left hilum is about 1 cm higher. Lingular pathology causes loss of clarity of the left heart border. The lower trachea is usually deviated to the right by the aorta.

74. A C D E

The volume of CO_2 produced in the body is less than the volume of O_2 consumed; expired minute volume is thus less than inspired volume. Although less oxygen will be carried dissolved in plasma at PO_2 70 mm Hg compared with PO_2 100 mm Hg, the great majority of oxygen is bound to haemoglobin, and this value will be almost unchanged (on the flat part of the dissociation curve). Arterial PO_2 is less than alveolar PO_2 due to inexact matching of ventilation to perfusion and the effects of anatomical right to left shunts. When the dissociation curve is right-shifted, a higher PO_2 is needed to produce the same degree of saturation of haemoglobin with oxygen, i.e. its oxygen affinity has fallen. Acidosis, a rise in temperature, and a rise in erythrocyte 2, 3 diphosphoglycerate concentration decrease affinity.

75. Sarcoidosis

A affects the lungs in about 25% of cases
B is associated with deficient B-lymphocyte mediated immunity
C is excluded by a negative Kveim test
D is often associated with a raised serum angiotensin converting enzyme (SACE) activity
E is associated with erythema marginatum

Your answers: A.........B.........C.........D.........E.........

76. Pleural calcification occurs in patients with a past medical history of

A occupational asbestos exposure
B haemothorax
C tuberculous pleural effusion
D working as a coal miner
E chickenpox pneumonia

Your answers: A.........B.........C.........D.........E.........

77. Acute bronchiolitis

A usually affects infants in the first year of life
B is most commonly caused by respiratory syncytial virus (RSV)
C characteristically, causes stridor
D causes crackles audible on auscultation as well as wheezes
E may cause sudden complete laryngeal obstruction if the throat is examined

Your answers: A.........B.........C.........D.........E.........

Answers overleaf

75. D

Sarcoidosis affects the lungs in 90% or more of patients in most reported series. It usually causes deficient T-lymphocyte mediated (cellular) immunity. About 25% of patients with sarcoidosis have a negative Kveim test; false positives are much rarer (1-2%). A high level of SACE activity probably indicates increased macrophage activity and thus active sarcoidosis; high levels are also found in Gaucher's disease and in leprosy and other granulomatous disorders. Erythema marginatum occurs in rheumatic fever, erythema nodosum may be associated with sarcoidosis.

76. A B C

Very extensive pleural calcification is likely to be due to old tuberculosis or haemothorax. Calcified pleural plaques may be difficult to see radiologically *en face*, but may be more readily visible along the lateral chest wall or on the diaphragmatic pleura. Oblique radiographs may help. Pleural calcification is not a feature of coal-workers' pneumoconiosis or chickenpox pneumonia; the latter may result in miliary calcification of the lung fields.

77. A B D

Neonates and older children usually have minimal symptoms of infection with RSV. The infection is very 'seasonal'; in Great Britain, almost all cases occur between December and May. Stridor is a feature of croup, not bronchiolitis. One cause of croup is acute epiglottitis, usually due to *Haemophilus influenzae*, in which examination of the throat may precipitate sudden complete obstruction.

78. There is a recognised association between pulmonary fibrosis and the following:

A psoriasis with arthropathy
B ankylosing spondylitis
C systemic sclerosis
D systemic lupus erythematosus
E sulphasalazine

Your answers: A.........B.........C.........D.........E.........

79. During an acute asthma attack

A alveolar-arterial PO_2 difference is increased
B functional residual capacity (FRC) is increased
C residual volume (RV) is decreased
D vital capacity (VC) is decreased
E arterial PCO_2 is usually normal or low

Your answers: A.........B.........C.........D.........E.........

80. Bronchiectasis

A is dilatation and destruction of airspaces distal to the terminal bronchioles
B may be complicated by life-threatening haemoptysis
C is often associated with infection by anaerobic bacteria
D has an association with dextrocardia
E affects the smaller bronchi in allergic bronchopulmonary aspergillosis

Your answers: A.........B.........C.........D.........E.........

Answers overleaf

78. B C D E

Pulmonary fibrosis in patients with ankylosing spondylitis is typically in the upper lobes and may mimic tuberculosis. Systemic sclerosis and systemic lupus erythematosus produce fibrosis, especially in the mid and lower zones, which is radiologically and clinically indistinguishable from cryptogenic fibrosing alveolitis. Sulphasalazine given for inflammatory bowel disease may cause pulmonary fibrosis; there is an independent association between inflammatory bowel disease itself and bronchiectasis.

79. A B D E

Perfusion of un-ventilated or under-ventilated areas of lung affected by airways closure or mucus plugging is effectively a 'shunt' of deoxygenated blood from right to left. The tendency to hypoxia enhances respiratory drive, keeping PCO_2 normal or low, but this is not the whole explanation; stimulation of airway receptors also plays a part. A rising arterial PCO_2 indicates fatigue and *is a very serious prognostic sign*; the patient may require mechanical ventilation. Asthmatics breathe at high lung volumes, tending to keep collapsing airways open; air trapping occurs distal to closed or plugged bronchi. FRC and RV are therefore high, while VC is reduced.

80. B C D

A is the definition of emphysema. Mild haemoptysis is common; severe haemoptysis occurs and can be fatal. Anaerobes are usually responsible if the sputum is foul tasting or strongly smelling. Ciliary abnormalities are responsible for Kartagener's syndrome of dextrocardia, bronchiectasis and absent or hypoplastic frontal sinuses. **Proximal** bronchiectasis is the usual consequence of repeated episodes of bronchial plugging by the tenacious secretions in allergic bronchopulmonary aspergillosis.

81. The following fungi may cause pulmonary disease:

A *Aspergillus fumigatus*
B *Aspergillus clavatus*
C *Malassezia furfur*
D *Trichophyton rubrum*
E *Cryptococcus neoformans*

Your answers: A.........B.........C.........D.........E.........

82. Pneumonia due to the following organisms frequently cavitates:

A *Streptococcus pneumoniae*
B *Staphylococcus aureus*
C *Klebsiella*
D *Mycobacterium tuberculosis*
E *Mycoplasma pneumoniae*

Your answers: A.........B.........C.........D.........E.........

83. The following statements are correct:

A the bronchial arteries usually arise directly from the aorta
B the visceral pleura is supplied by branches of the bronchial arteries
C lymphatic drainage from the left lung is via the thoracic duct
D the visceral pleura is innervated only by autonomic fibres
E all bronchi have cartilage in their walls

Your answers: A........B........C........D........E........

Answers overleaf

81. A B E

A. fumigatus is the most common fungus to cause pulmonary disease in Great Britain. The three main clinical syndromes are: 1. allergic bronchopulmonary aspergillosis, with wheezing, fever, eosinophilia and pulmonary infiltration; 2. aspergilloma, a fungus ball in a pre-existing pulmonary cavity; 3. invasive aspergillosis in immunosuppressed patients. *A. clavatus* causes extrinsic allergic alveolitis (malt-worker's lung). *Cryptococcus* usually affects immunosuppressed patients and may cause a variety of radiographic appearances. Fungi C and D cause skin disease (pityriasis versicolor and tinea pedis, respectively).

82. B C D

Str. pneumoniae classically causes a lobar pneumonia; cavitation is unusual. *Staph. aureus* often produces abscesses which can look like thin-walled cysts. These may rupture into the pleura to give a pneumothorax, a complication commoner in children than adults. *Klebsiella* often causes a lobar pneumonia with cavitation; upper lobes are commonly affected. Patients with *Staphylococcus* or *Klebsiella* pneumonia are usually extremely ill. A clinically well patient with a normal chest X-ray and *Staphylococcus* or *Klebsiella* in their sputum does not have pneumonia due to these organisms and usually requires no specific treatment.

83. A B C D E

Occasionally, bronchial arteries arise from or communicate with intercostal, subclavian or internal mammary arteries; more usually they arise direct from the aorta. Parietal pleura receives its blood supply from the intercostal arteries. Lymph drains into systemic veins at the subclavian/internal jugular junction via the right lymphatic duct on the right and the thoracic duct on the left. Parietal pleura is innervated by spinal, intercostal and phrenic nerves. All airways with cartilage in their walls are called bronchi; distal smaller airways with no cartilage are called bronchioles.

84. In the treatment of tuberculosis

A enlargement of tuberculous glands during treatment indicates a resistant organism
B tuberculous pleural effusions usually resolve with chemotherapy alone
C 6 months' treatment with appropriate antituberculous drugs is usually sufficient
D rifampicin may be associated with ocular toxicity
E isoniazid may be associated with peripheral neuropathy

Your answers: A.........B.........C.........D.........E.........

85. In a pleural effusion

A glucose content of the fluid is often low in rheumatoid disease
B amylase may be high in acute pancreatitis
C malignant cells are present in almost all cases due to malignancy
D blood staining is virtually pathognomonic of malignancy
E about 100 ml of fluid must be present before it is detectable on the chest radiograph

Your answers: A.........B.........C.........D.........E.........

86. The following statements are correct:

A salbutamol may precipitate premature labour
B streptomycin causes VIIIth cranial nerve damage
C *Haemophilus influenzae* is rarely resistant to amoxycillin
D *Pseudomonas aeruginosa* is usually sensitive to cotrimoxazole
E erythromycin is excreted principally by the liver

Your answers: A.........B.........C.........D.........E.........

Answers overleaf

84. B C E

Enlargement of tuberculous nodes and appearance of new nodes during treatment is due to an ill-understood immunological reaction and occurs in up to one third of cases. Treatment with 4 drugs (including rifampicin and pyrazinamide) for 2 months followed by 4 months on two drugs (including rifampicin) is effective treatment. It is likely, although not yet generally accepted, that an initial 3 drugs (including rifampicin and pyrazinamide) is sufficient. Ethambutol, not rifampicin, causes ocular toxicity. Peripheral neuropathy with isoniazid is commoner in 'slow acetylators' but now rare with standard doses. In those requiring higher doses (e.g. TB meningitis), pyridoxine 10 mg daily reduces the risk of neuropathy.

85. A B

Pleural fluid glucose is often low in rheumatoid disease, in effusion due to infection, and when large numbers of malignant cells are present. Malignant cells are found in 50% or less of pleural effusions due to malignancy. Bloodstaining occurs in effusions other than those caused by malignancy, particularly pulmonary embolism. Several hundred ml of fluid must be present before radiological visualisation is possible.

86. B E

Salbutamol has been used in the treatment of premature labour. Plasma streptomycin levels should be monitored to avoid VIIIth nerve damage. About 20-40% of strains of *H. influenzae* are ß-lactamase producing. *Ps. aeruginosa* is usually sensitive to aminoglycosides, to penicillin derivatives like carbenicillin, azlocillin and ticarcillin, and to some cephalosporins. Care should be exercised in prescribing erythromycin to patients with liver dysfunction; occasionally, cholestatic jaundice has been reported.

87. In patients with obstructive sleep apnoea syndrome, there is an increased incidence of the following:

A systemic hypertension
B pulmonary hypertension
C daytime somnolence
D polycythaemia
E depression

Your answers: A.........B.........C.........D.........E.........

88. There is an increased risk of pneumothorax associated with

A menstruation
B pulmonary tuberculosis
C staphylococcal pneumonia
D cystic fibrosis
E Marfan's syndrome

Your answers: A.........B.........C.........D.........E.........

89. Pleural effusion may be due to

A hepatic abscess
B acute pancreatitis
C oesophageal perforation
D myocardial infarction without left ventricular failure
E coal-workers' pneumoconiosis

Your answers: A.........B.........C.........D.........E.........

Answers overleaf

87. A B C D E

The systemic hypertension often seen in patients with obstructive sleep apnoea is poorly understood. Pulmonary hypertension and secondary polycythaemia are thought to result from the hypoxaemia that accompanies the episodes of apnoea, and which in some individuals may persist during waking hours. Daytime somnolence is characteristic; patients may fall asleep whilst driving, eating or talking. Depression affects at least 25% of patients.

88. A B C D E

Almost all pulmonary diseases are associated with some increased risk of pneumothorax, albeit very small in most conditions. Catamenial pneumothorax is uncommon but well described; opinions differ as to its relationship with intrathoracic endometriosis. Pneumothorax complicating staphylococcal pneumonia is commoner in children than adults. Acute deterioration in cystic fibrosis (and, indeed, any other pulmonary illness) should always raise the suspicion of pneumothorax.

89. A B C D

Hepatic abscesses, pyogenic or amoebic, may be associated with pleural effusion. About 15% of patients with acute pancreatitis have a pleural effusion; the exudate resulting from pancreatic inflammation is probably transported across the diaphragm in lymphatics which leak the fluid (containing high levels of pancreatic enzymes) into the pleural space. Pancreatic pseudocysts may develop a direct sinus between pancreas and pleural space. About 60% of patients with oesophageal perforations have a pleural effusion. Pleural effusion may occur in 'post-cardiac injury syndrome' (Dressler's syndrome), usually due to myocardial infarction, but also occurring after cardiac surgery and blunt chest trauma.

90. Adult respiratory distress syndrome (ARDS) may complicate

A septicaemia
B aspiration of gastric contents
C multiple blood transfusions
D near-drowning
E prolonged hypotension

Your answers: A.........B.........C.........D.........E.........

91. *Bordetella pertussis* **infections**

A are characteristically associated with fever
B usually cause a lymphocytosis
C may be complicated by pneumothorax
D are diagnosed by the demonstration of a rising antibody titre
E may be vaccinated against with live, attenuated organisms

Your answers: A.........B.........C.........D.........E.........

92. In a 10-year-old girl

A a positive Heaf (tuberculin) test indicates immunity to tuberculosis
B repeated chest infections are likely to be due to chronic bronchitis
C inhaled corticosteroids are contraindicated as treatment for asthma
D asthma is usually associated with positive skin prick tests to common allergens
E cystic fibrosis may be diagnosed for the first time

Your answers: A.........B.........C.........D.........E.........

Answers overleaf

90. A B C D E

ARDS is characterised by pulmonary oedema of non-cardiogenic origin and may result from a wide range of insults. Complement-mediated aggregation of leucocytes in the lungs, with subsequent release of substances resulting in endothelial damage has usually been regarded as the responsible mechanism, but latterly this has been questioned. The lungs are stiff and non-compliant and patients may be very difficult to ventilate. Corticosteroids have little or no effect on the progress of the disease once the full clinical picture is established.

91. B C

B. pertussis causes the clinical illness usually referred to as whooping cough. Fever is not a feature unless secondary bacterial infection supervenes. Pneumothorax, subcutaneous and mediastinal emphysema, rectal prolapse and inguinal hernia may result from the paroxysms of coughing. Diagnosis is made by isolation of organisms from nasopharyngeal swabs (formerly by the 'cough plate' technique). Pertussis vaccine is a killed preparation, usually given with diphtheria and tetanus toxoid (triple vaccine) in a series of three injections beginning at age 6 to 12 weeks. A booster dose is given prior to school entry.

92. D E

A positive tuberculin test indicates previous exposure to antigen, *not* immunity. If this is not due to previous BCG vaccination (usually given at age 13-14) specialist chest assessment is necessary. Repeated chest infections are almost certainly due to undiagnosed asthma or, much less commonly, an underlying immune deficiency; consider also inhaled foreign body. Inhaled corticosteroids in standard doses are safe and effective. Most asthmatic 10 year olds are atopic (i.e. have positive skin prick tests). Cystic fibrosis is not always diagnosed in infancy; mildly affected patients in particular may present throughout childhood and adolescence and even as adults.

93. The syndrome of inappropriate antidiuretic hormone (ADH) secretion may be associated with

A tuberculosis
B chronic bronchitis
C carcinoma of the bronchus
D lung abscess
E emphysema

Your answers: A.........B.........C.........D.........E.........

94. In normal individuals

A the right lung is larger than the left
B the lingula is anatomically part of the left lower lobe
C the terminal bronchioles lead into the alveolar ducts
D alveoli are functionally distinct, without collateral ventilation
E the glottis widens during inspiration

Your answers: A.........B.........C.........D.........E.........

95. The following tests or measurements will help distinguish a patient with upper airways (laryngeal or tracheal) obstruction from one with asthma:

A peak expiratory flow rate (PEFR)
B ratio of forced expiratory volume in first second (FEV_1) to forced vital capacity (FVC)
C flow/volume loop
D bronchoscopy
E total lung capacity (TLC)

Your answers: A.........B.........C.........D.........E.........

Answers overleaf

93. A C D

Carcinoma of the bronchus, most commonly small cell anaplastic (oat cell) carcinoma is the commonest intrathoracic cause of inappropriate ADH secretion. Extrathoracic neoplastic causes include tumours of pancreas, prostate, colon and nasopharynx, and lymphomas. Central nervous system infections, trauma and space occupying lesions may also be responsible.

94. A E

The position of the heart and differing bronchial anatomy means that the right lung is usually larger than the left. The lingula is part of the left upper lobe. Terminal bronchioles lead into respiratory bronchioles, which in turn lead into alveolar ducts. Collateral ventilation takes place between alveoli via the pores of Kohn. There is active, neurally mediated widening of the glottic aperture during inspiration.

95. C D

PEFR and FEV_1 to FVC ratio will be low in both asthma and upper airways obstruction. The two tests **together** may be useful, since in upper airways obstruction PEFR is usually (but not always) disproportionately reduced compared with FEV_1. FEV_1 (ml) divided by PEFR (l/min) is usually less than 10. Values greater than 10 are very suggestive of large airways obstruction. Inspection of typical flow/volume loops, the best physiological test for distinguishing asthma from upper airways obstruction, will help explain why this is the case.

96. The following may be due to rheumatoid disease:

A pleural effusion
B fibrosing alveolitis
C rheumatoid nodules in the lungs
D stridor
E haemoptysis

Your answers: A.........B.........C.........D.........E.........

97. Haemoptysis may be a feature of the following conditions:

A tricuspid stenosis
B Goodpasture's syndrome
C aspergilloma
D allergic bronchopulmonary aspergillosis
E asbestosis

Your answers: A.........B.........C.........D.........E.........

98. The following statements are correct concerning a metabolic acidosis:

A arterial PCO_2 is high
B plasma bicarbonate is low
C arterial PO_2 is normal or high
D haemoglobin releases oxygen more readily in the tissues
E hypokalaemia may occur

Your answers: A.........B.........C.........D.........E.........

Answers overleaf

96. A B C D

Pleural thickening and effusion are the commonest forms of rheumatoid lung disease. Rheumatoid nodules are rare. Rheumatoid fibrosing alveolitis is clinically and radiologically indistinguishable from the cryptogenic form; some histological differences may be found. Rheumatoid arthritis may ankylose the cricoarytenoid joints, resulting in hoarseness and stridor. This possibility should be considered in any patient with rheumatoid arthritis who presents with 'asthma'.

97. B C

Mitral stenosis may result in haemoptysis due to the high left atrial pressure and pulmonary congestion. Goodpasture's syndrome, due to anti- basement membrane antibodies, affects glomeruli and lungs, classically causing haemoptysis and nephritis. Aspergillomata may cause severe bronchiectasis if they erode into an adjacent pulmonary or, particularly, bronchial vessel.

98. B C D

The high H^+ concentration in a metabolic acidosis stimulates the respiratory centre and hyperventilation occurs; arterial PO_2 thus tends to be high and PCO_2 is low. Bicarbonate buffer is used up and plasma bicarbonate falls; the carbonic acid generated by this process is itself buffered initially by haemoglobin and subsequently leads to increased CO_2 output by the lungs. Acidosis shifts the oxygen dissociation curve of haemoglobin to the right (i.e. affinity falls). At tissue PO_2 the haemoglobin can carry less oxygen than formerly and more is given up to the tissues. Acidosis shifts potassium from intracellular to extracellular compartments. Urinary excretion of K^+ increases, so patients may be whole-body K^+ depleted despite having a high plasma K^+.

99. The following statements are correct concerning a respiratory acidosis:

A acutely, pH and plasma bicarbonate fall
B renal excretion of bicarbonate increases
C the affinity of haemoglobin for oxygen is decreased
D arterial PCO_2 remains normal
E cerebral blood flow increases

Your answers: A.........B.........C.........D.........E.........

00. Causes of pulmonary hypertension include

A systemic sclerosis
B chronic salicylate ingestion
C kyphoscoliosis
D long-term residence at an altitude of 4000 metres
E pulmonary veno-occlusive disease

Your answers: A.........B.........C.........D.........E.........

Answers overleaf

99. B C E

The cause of a respiratory acidosis is a high arterial PCO_2. Since 70% of CO_2 is carried in the blood as bicarbonate, pH falls and bicarbonate increases. Renal compensation occurs with increased excretion of bicarbonate, levels of bicarbonate thus returning towards normal after a few days. Acidosis (respiratory *or* metabolic) shifts the oxygen dissociation curve of haemoglobin to the right, i.e. affinity of haemoglobin for oxygen is decreased. Cerebral vessels are dilated by a high PCO_2; papilloedema and cerebral oedema may occur.

100. A C D E

Systemic sclerosis causes pulmonary fibrosis and obliteration of pulmonary capillaries; larger vessels show medial hyperplasia and intimal proliferation, narrowing the lumen. Kyphoscoliosis with consequent alveolar hypoventilation (particularly during sleep) will, like high altitude residence and any other cause of alveolar hypoxia, lead to hypoxic pulmonary vasoconstriction and eventually structural vascular changes and sustained pulmonary hypertension. Pulmonary veno-occlusive disease is, like plexogenic pulmonary hypertension, a cause of so-called ‘primary pulmonary hypertension’.

REVISION INDEX

Each item in this index refers to a specific question or answer. The numbers given refer to question numbers not page numbers.